A QIN BOWEI ANTHOLOGY

CLINICAL ESSAYS

BY MASTER PHYSICIAN QIN BOWEI

Translated and Edited by

Charles Chace

and

Zhang Ting Liang

Paradigm Publications   **1997**   **Brookline, Massachusetts**

A Qin Bowei Anthology
Clinical Essays
by Master Physician Qin Bowei

translated and edited by

Charles Chace and Zhang Ting Liang

Library of Congress Cataloging-in-Publication Data:

Ch'in, Po-wei.
A Qin Bowei anthology : clinical essays by Master Physician Qin
Bowei / translated and edited by Charles Chace and Zhang Ting Liang.
    p. cm.
Translated from Chinese.
Includes bibliographical references and index.
ISBN 0-912111-41-0 (pbk.)
1. Medicine, Chinese. I. Chace, Charles, 1958-. II. Liang, Zhang Ting, 1955-.
III. Title.
R601.C48215 1997
615.5'3'0951--dc21   97-4783
                                             CIP

Paradigm Publications

44 Linden Street

Brookline, Massachusetts 02146 U.S.A.

TABLE OF CONTENTS

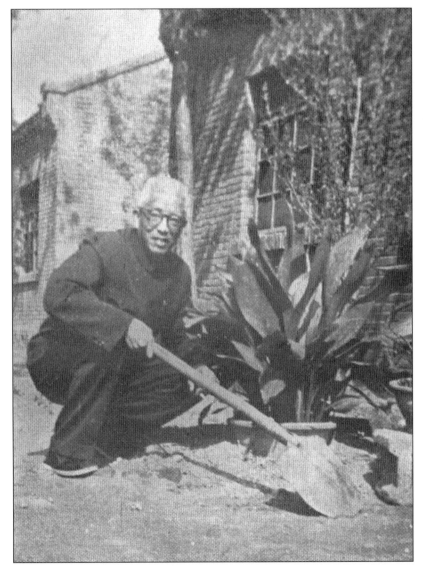

Qin Bowei in his garden

DEDICATION

This book is dedicated to my father Charles W. Chace, M.D., who taught me a thing or two about doctoring in spite of himself.

ACKNOWLEDGEMENTS

I would like to thank the following people for their invaluable input on this project over the last ten years. Bob Felt, Bob Flaws, Nigel Wiseman, Dan Bensky, Sharon Weizenbaum, Yang Shou-zhong, Andy Ellis, and Honora Wolfe have saved me from untold embarrassments. This anthology never would have seen the light of day without their help. Be that as it may, any errors are my own.

DESIGNATION

Paradigm Publications is a participant in the Council of Oriental Medical Publishers (C.O.M.P.) and supports their effort to make readers aware of the sources of East Asian medical information and the methods used to represent it in English. By C.O.M.P. guidelines, this work is a "denotive translation."

The translation is based upon the *English-Chinese–Chinese-English Dictionary of Chinese Medicine,* by Nigel Wiseman, published by the Hunan Science and Technology Press, Hunan, China, 1995.

The medical substance and formula nomenclature are direct translations of the Chinese based on the methods and terms of the translational glossary. The Chinese is represented by toned Pinyin, which, while not absolutely unique due to homophones, does permit direct reference to the source text. In addition, an English translation is provided, typically in parentheses. These translations are the common names found in unabridged English dictionaries. If there is no common name, the name by which the agent is known in commerce, for example, by botanists or agriculturalists, is used. For substances where no English name is in use, names have been structured according to the same principles. When part of an English substance name is enclosed in square brackets - [ ] - that part is optional. That is, although that part of the name may be used in English works, it is not required to uniquely identify the substance in the 5,600 agent materia medica of the *Chinese Medical Dictionary* of the People's Republic of China.

Because Qin Bowei's work is also of interest to sinologists and linguists, and for the benefit of Western clinicians who are studying medical Chinese, textual interpolations have been noted to a greater extent than modern editorial style requires.

TRANSLATOR'S INTRODUCTION

It is virtually impossible for any student of Chinese medicine to complete his or her education without at least gaining a passing familiarity with Zhāng Zhòngjǐng, Zhōu Dānxī, Lǐ Shízhēn, and the other architects of Chinese medicine who lived and worked during the last two millennia. However, in the West most students of Chinese medicine have had little or no exposure to the twentieth century Chinese thinkers and practitioners who have defined T.C.M. as it is known in China today. They are the architects of the most recent additions to the edifice of Chinese medicine.

QIN BOWEI'S PLACE IN HISTORY

Tradition is venerated every bit as much in Chinese medicine as it is in Asian cultures in general. Mere modern innovations have been regarded with a certain disdain as the ancients were seen as the source of "Truth." This trend, although particularly pronounced during the Sung, Jin, and Yuan periods, is pervasive in Chinese history and seems to be balanced by epochal book burnings and cultural erasures. One of the many difficulties such a perspective currently creates for Westerners is that we have neither access to the most basic pre-modern sources nor an appreciation of the overall development of Chinese medical ideas. Thus most of us are forced to rely on interpretations of T.C.M. provided by Western clinicians, which, while often useful, further remove us from a broader view of T.C.M. Fortunately, articulate interpretations of T.C.M. have been provided by twentieth century physicians in the Peoples' Republic of China and it is to these viewpoints that we may turn to seek an essential link between pre-modern sources and present Western conceptions of Chinese medicine.

At the beginning of the twentieth century there were two opposed political and philosophical trends that affected the course of medical practice in China. The first was the desire to purge Chinese society of all the superstitious, irrational, politically incorrect, and unscientific practices of the "old China." Of these, Chinese medicine was among the most prominent. On the other hand, fearing they would be seen as totally surrendering to the West, government leaders wanted to maintain a Chinese cultural identity in the face of an ever-growing Western scientism. Each of these trends gained ascendency at different times during the first half of the twentieth century.

As early as the Guomintang government, a resolution was passed completely forbidding the practice of Chinese medicine in China. This event forced a wide range of divergent factions in Chinese medicine to come together to meet the challenge of oppression rather than bickering among themselves over points of theory. The National Institute of Medicine *[Guó Yī Guǎn]* was founded to defend indigenous medicine against further threats. Professional medical associations, research centers, hospitals, and schools developed from this common interest. In their effort to present Chinese medicine as something more cohesive than a bag of unrelated clinical and theoretical tricks, these associations sowed the seeds that would produce the homogenous blend of styles we know today as "Traditional Chinese Medicine," or T.C.M.

By the early 1950's, the Communist government of China had embraced Chinese medicine as a means of caring for a population of more than a half billion people. Initially, this was an emergency method only intended to serve until more biomedical physicians could be trained and a modern medical infrastructure established. This goal gradually evolved because Chinese medicine retained popularity relative to its Western rival. This homogenization of Chinese medicine continued through the 1960's, including, as a notable example, the standardization of the patterns that comprise T.C.M. today. Committees based in colleges and hospitals decided what was part of Chinese medicine and what was not. These decisions were directly influenced by a political climate that was in constant flux. For example, those aspects of Chinese medicine dealing with chronobiology *(zī wǔ liú chù)* enjoyed periods of great interest and suffered periods where they were considered anathemas. The study of the application of the *Yì Jīng* to medical practice is another prominent example of a subject buffeted by the whims of political doctrine.

Efforts to forge an integration of Chinese and Western medicine ultimately made Chinese medicine subservient to Western medicine. The theoretical basis of Chinese medicine was gradually abandoned in favor of empirical tools that could be quickly learned and used by "barefoot doctors." However, by the 1970's and 1980's, led by writers like Qin Bowei, there was a resurgence of interest in Chinese medicine as an entire system, not just a bag of clinical tricks to be dusted-off and polished by science.

In these essays, Qin's emphasis on the intellectual process of Chinese medicine is fairly understood as an argument against this erosion of the theoretical foundations of Chinese medicine. As such, these essays are a part of Chinese medicine rarely seen in the West, elements of its accommodation not only to Chinese social and political demands but to the modern Western approach to human health that predominates in China. Thus, his writings provide the reader with not only the depth of detail but also the scope of medical discussions in China, an aspect of China's indigenous medicine that is lacking in the official T.C.M. texts the Chinese government produces for export to the West.

THE CLINICAL PERSPECTIVE

The virtues of Chinese medicine in treating patients in a manner that is comprehensive yet unique to the individual are widely acknowledged.

That the practice of Chinese medicine is itself very individualized is often taken for granted and is therefore rarely considered in Western books or schools. However, in the clinic, Chinese medicine is an instrument that each practitioner plays differently, some better than others, and each with an individual prediliction for a theoretical or therapeutic style that best suits their individual skills and personality. This is what breathes life into the tradition of Chinese medicine and allows it to grow.

Even in the West, despite the narrowed scope imposed by license-testing committees and their profound influence on T.C.M. education in the United States, no two practitioners practice identically. The general Western perception of a monolithic T.C.M. orthodoxy is an illusion reinforced because there are so few T.C.M. texts available in English that are actual translations of Chinese works. In the perspective of history, the ground rules of T.C.M. are agreed upon just as the shape of an instrument is fixed. Yet, it is how that instrument is fashioned by the craftsman and played by the practitioner that ultimately determines the quality of the music.

In terms of the Chinese medical writings, the aspect of practice that is individual is most strongly represented in three interrelated branches of this literature. These are: case histories *(yī àn)*, medical discussions *(yī huà)*, and medical theses *(yī lùn)*. Case histories are a complete record of a patient's history, symptoms, and signs, as well as the diagnosis, the therapeutic methods selected, and the drugs prescribed by the physician. At present, few examples of the case history literature are available in English. Anthologies of case histories such as *Fleshing Out The Bones*[1] and *Acupuncture Case Histories From China*[2] are not only few but play a negligible role in Western acupuncture education, particularly in relation to their importance in China. Qin Bowei has written extensively on the importance of case histories in the practice of T.C.M. and a translation of his essay on that topic appears in *Fleshing Out the Bones.*[3] His essay on water swelling in this collection is an excellent example of his approach to recording case histories and how they may be used as a platform for a medical discussion. Qin's essay on supplementation, because it further develops and presents his personal ideas of that topic, takes the form of a medical discussion.

Medical discussions have no fixed form but usually include records of a doctor's personal ideas, successful cases, the experience of self and others, as well as research concerning medical problems. These are essentially a physician's notes on the study of medicine. Medical theses are works consisting of the doctor's personal ideas and are equivalent to contemporary medical theses. The majority of essays in this collection are medical theses. Again, few theses and discussions have made their way into English. Although they are likely to be found in professional periodicals if anywhere, medical theses and discussions have not as yet found a significant place in Western education or intra-professional communications.

---

[1]Chace, Charles, tr., *Fleshing Out the Bones*, Boulder, CO:Blue Poppy Press, 1992.

[2]Chen Ji-rui and Nissi Wang, ed., *Acupuncture Case Histories from China*, Seattle WA: Eastland Press, 1988.

[3]Chace, Charles, tr., *Fleshing Out the Bones, op. cit.*

Xú Dàchūn's essays as translated by Paul Unschuld in *Forgotten Traditions of Ancient Chinese Medicine*[4] are an example of the classical genre. Bob Flaws is one of the few Western writers to have adopted these traditional formats and his journal essays are contemporary examples of their genre.

In all three classes of writing, even the most theoretical dissertations permit authors to articulate their biases and individual inclinations. In practice, case histories, medical discussions, and medical theses overlap. For example, case histories may form the bulk of a medical discussion, or a case history may be used simply as a point of departure for a long commentary. What is common to all these forms is that Chinese medicine is viewed through the individual's perspective. This is not Chinese medicine by committee. It is, on the contrary, a richer and often more idiosyncratic view of a specific condition or disharmony. Individual variations in the manner of applying Chinese medical principles are also brought to light.

The clinical writings of individual physicians comprise a significant part of the corpus of contemporary medical literature. Anthologies of essays and discussions by well-known modern doctors are abundant as are collections of case histories. These case histories are arranged in a variety of ways. They may cover a specific area of medicine such as gynecology or they may be arranged by geographic locales. There is, for example, a fine anthology of case histories from eminent Shanghai doctors.[5] Writings such as these provide an immediate clinical reference to empirically proven approaches for a vast range of illnesses.

Also inherent in modern Chinese medical writings is a lack of ambiguity. An author's meaning is often more clearly articulated in a modern text than in a similar pre-modern one. There is a premium on clarity even at the expense of literary style, a feature that may be observed in the accompanying essays. This makes these modern works all the more accessible. Even given substantial cultural differences between East and West, the issues addressed by modern Chinese writers more closely approximate the concerns of Western readers.

THE WRITINGS OF QIN BOWEI

Qin Bowei was one of the most respected physicians of twentieth century China, not only as a clinician but also as a writer and educator. Of the many master physicians in the Peoples Republic of China, Qin Bowei was unique in the scope of his activities. In addition to clinical work, he wrote extensively on Chinese medicine and founded a number of colleges of T.C.M. He was active politically in insuring the perpetuation of T.C.M. when the Guomintang regime repressed Chinese medicine. He then served the health ministry of the P.R.C. in an administrative capacity during the 1950's.

[4]Unschuld, Paul U., *Forgotten Traditions of Ancient Chinese Medicine, The I-hsueh Yuan Lun of 1757 by Hsu Ta-ch'un,* Brookline, MA: Paradigm Publications, 1990.

[5]Shanghai Hygiene Bureau, ed., *Shanghai Lao Zhong Yi Jing Shan Shi Pian,* Shanghai: Shanghai Science and Technology Press, 1978.

The writings of Qin Bowei reflect both the full rigor of the T.C.M. approach and an astonishing fluidity in its clinical execution. In Qin Bowei we see an old world Chinese doctor fluently articulating himself within the framework of modern T.C.M. – the paradigm that he helped to define. Included in this anthology is a broad sampling of Qin Bowei's writings, including formal essays such as those on liver disorders and the life gate, as well as case histories and lecture notes. A memoriam written by two of his more illustrious students as an introduction to the anthology from which these essays were excerpted has also been included to frame his medical accomplishments in the context of his life. This elicits a more meaningful picture of Qin's life than raw biographical data.

Qin Bowei's essay on liver disorders forms the centerpiece of this collection. It is a step by step analysis of the rational process inherent in T.C.M., beginning with a defining of terms and concluding with the modification of prescriptions. I believe that this is the most comprehensive discussion of liver patterns available in English at this time. Qin Bowei asserts that there can be no real discussion of liver disorders – or Chinese medicine at all for that matter – until we have defined our terminology. This he has done in exquisite detail. His use of precise terminology throughout the diagnostic and therapeutic process reflects a degree of intellectual rigor found in few contemporary authors. This is so much the case that one would be tempted to dismiss such details as his personal taste had their clinical value not been so aptly revealed.

Qin Bowei's differentiation between liver qi and liver depression is a case in point. In currently available English treatment manuals, these two liver patterns are essentially indistinguishable. Yet, when applied to treatment, Qin's discrimination provides a clarity that can clearly determine whether or not a patient's therapy will succeed or fail. For example, intrinsic to liver qi is the presence of horizontal counterflow and a hyperactivity of the liver's capacity for coursing and draining. Liver depression, on the other hand, is characterized by a failure of the liver's capacity for coursing and draining. While the symptoms may be similar, they are exactly opposite in effect. Without the definition of distinct treatment methods for each pattern, and the terminological refinement required to label those distinctions, success in treatment will be no better than random.

Of equal utility is Qin's clarification of redundant treatment measures that have identical implications. For instance, he flatly states that balancing the liver, draining the liver, and coursing the liver all mean the same thing. The clarification of such redundancies is no less important than the description of the clinical nuances found in terminological detail.

As a reader of a wide variety of contemporary Chinese authors it is clear to me that many writers exercise greater latitude in their use of Chinese terminology. However, as a practitioner viewing Qin's perspectives in the light of clinical practice, I am impressed by the clarity Qin's rigor brings to every step of the diagnostic process. Qin's precision clarifies even the choice of individual medicinals in a prescription. The internal consistency of his perspective is evident from start to finish. T.C.M. is a difficult instrument to play, especially difficult, it would seem, for Western students who, in utilizing the fluidity of the system, fall easy prey to sloppy thinking. Qin's dissertation on liver disorders addresses this issue incisively. The material in the discussion on liver disorders has been summarized in table form at the end of each section to provide for easy access and cross-referencing.

The chapter on prescription composition is clearly a reworking of lecture notes. It is, however, a lucid and articulate discussion of the many considerations that are involved in composing a prescription and, again, among the most detailed essays available in English. He often instructs by example, comparing the strengths and weaknesses of such masters as Zhāng Zhòngjǐng, Lǐ Dōngyuán and Yè Tiānshì. For example, it is Zhāng Zhòngjǐng who Qin considered foremost in organizing a prescription. However he also acknowledged that the precision of Lǐ Dōngyuán's medicinal combinations was inspired. It is in this essay that Qin Bowei voices his opinions regarding *Yín Qiào Sǎn* (Lonicera and Forsythia Formula), the famous prescription for resolving external wind heat that is paradoxically named after two medicinals specifically aimed at clearing toxic heat.[6]

Mìng mén [life gate] as a concept has attracted a fair bit of interest in the recent acupuncture literature. Matsumoto and Birch's *Hara Diagnosis, Reflections on the Sea,* provides the most comprehensive treatment of life gate in English to date. However, the clinical utility of the life gate in herbal medicine has not been so carefully addressed. In Qin's essay, "Preliminary Inquiry into the Life Gate" we see an herbalist's understanding of life gate both in theoretical terms and as clinical ramifications for prescription. Many of the most familiar prescriptions for kidney patterns are differentiated here. Some of this material has been summarized in the appendices of *Scatology and the Gate of Life.*[7] Qin Bowei's essay is here translated in its entirety.

It is always interesting to see how a writer deals with an individual symptom. In perhaps the most theoretical discussion in this anthology, Qin Bowei addresses the issue of fever. Outlined in this work are sixteen distinct patterns that can give rise to fever and the methods for addressing each. Given the prevalence of fevers in the context of immune disorders and complex illnesses such as Epstein-Barr syndrome and post viral syndrome, Qin's essay offers a timely perspective.

Qin Bowei's essays on cough and water swelling are by contrast more clinical. The piece on water swelling is, in particular, arranged in essentially a note-taking format. Nonetheless, in his discussion of two cases of water swelling, Qin delineates between root and branch treatment measures at each stage of therapy. Also evident is a progression of treatment which is not so neat and tidy. Clarity here can be appreciated by anyone who has ever "lost the thread" in the midst of a complex and convoluted case. In Qin's "Brief Discussion of Supplementation," he, like many physicians before him, addresses the relative popularity of supplementing foods and medicinals and their relative value in medicine. Given that it is the

---

[6]Bensky and Barolet cite Qin Bowei's viewpoint in their discussion of *Yín Qiào Sǎn* in Barolet, Randall and Bensky, D., *Chinese Herbal Medicine, Formulas and Strategies,* Seattle, WA: Eastland Press, 1991.

[7]Flaws, Bob, *Scatology and the Gate of Life,* Boulder, CO: Blue Poppy Press, 1990.

panacea-like reputation of the mislabeled "tonic herbs" that most colors public perception of Chinese herbalism, the essay is both useful and timely.

Finally, a selection of case histories by Qin Bowei has been included. As a number of these pertain to edema, they integrate well with his essay on water swelling. It was somewhat disappointing that, given Qin Bowei's advocacy for publishing cases that had failed or gone poorly, I was unable to locate any record of his own clinical failures. These would, no doubt, be instructive. Be that as it may, in keeping with Qin's criteria for case histories, this selection of his own cases covers a broad spectrum of illness, both common and obscure, and offers ample evidence that he practiced what he preached.

NOTES ON THE TRANSLATION

Qin Bowei's essays have been translated in a manner as closely approaching the style of the original Chinese as possible. Some of the chapters read more like lecture notes than formal essays and we have attempted to retain this variety while still presenting a readable text. There are also certain proforma statements in the writings of the 1950's, 1960's, and 1970's that reflect the political climate prevailing in the Peoples' Republic at that time. Qin Bowei's requests for criticism and comment should be seen in this light, although his writings are for the most part mercifully free of "party-speak."

Qin was writing for practitioners, thus even when discussing the most fundamental aspects of liver disorders there is an assumption of essential familiarity with the basic structure of Chinese medical theory. Despite the close look we get at Qin Bowei's approach to medicine in these essays, this is not a "how to" book. The material is best ruminated upon and digested slowly. Its translation into one's own clinical practice comes from a widening of perspective rather than from the extraction of some neat formula from a particular page. Nonetheless, the material has been organized in a manner we hope will serve quick reference.

It is entirely possible for an acupuncturist to be oriented clinically, to the exclusion of scholarly endeavor. To a large extent this is because acupuncturists can more immediately benefit from learning to better manipulate qi than from reading books. However, Chinese herbal medicine is intimately tied to its literature. Familiarity with its development and the work of its major thinkers throughout history can only enhance clinical competence. If, for example, we compare two modern English translations based on the same approach such as *Acupuncture, a Comprehensive Text* and *Chinese Herbal Medicine, Formulas and Strategies,* we see much greater attention paid to historical context in the latter text. This is the result of the subject matter, despite the fact that both books are essentially clinical manuals.

It is my feeling that a clear understanding of the historical development of clinical ideas is essential to the practice of Chinese herbal medicine in the West. A characteristic of most Chinese T.C.M. writers is frequent references to pre-modern sources that are used to illustrate or justify a point. Qin Bowei is no stranger to this habit and his citations are edifying as they often reveal some unvisited region of the Chinese medical landscape.

A number of writers have made the point that the traditional forms of medicine practiced in China are not a homogenous entity but a heterogenous mixture of diverse influences such as shamanism and folk medicine as well as the theoretical systems familiar to most modern acupuncturists. Be that as it may, the phrase *zhòng yī*, or "Chinese medicine" as it appears in most modern medical writings, and Qin Bowei's are no exception, refers exclusively to what is today called "Traditional Chinese Medicine" and its direct ancestors. While modern physicians may acknowledge the existence of shamanic and demonological strains of healing, for whatever reasons, political or otherwise, they are not currently regarded as "Chinese medicine."

The essays in this anthology have been translated from *Qin Bo Wei Yi Wen Ji,* which was published in 1981 by Hunan Science and Technology Press. I am indebted to Bob Flaws for the extended loan of this text as it is no longer in print. Qin Bowei's case histories were excerpted from *Zhong Guo Xian Dai Ming Zhong Yi Yi An Jing Hua,* a collection of case studies by modern masters of Chinese medicine published by Beijing Press in 1990.

The translation system developed by Nigel Wiseman had been used throughout the text. As this translation makes use of the considerable conceptual breadth of that method, many of the clinical concepts and details may be unfamiliar to English readers. Definitions for terms that are not self evident have been footnoted and translator's annotations are present also where clarification of the text was in order, or I simply could not resist comment.

Charles Chace

Boulder, Colorado 1996

BIOGRAPHY OF QIN BOWEI

At 8.00 p.m. on January 27, 1970, in a ward of Dong Zhimen Hospital in Beijing, a grey haired, emaciated old man said with profound emotion, 'Death is inevitable. Death is not horrifying. However, my failure to pass on all my experiences in the study of T.C.M. is my eternal regret. I hope you. . ." The sound of the words diminished [becoming inaudible] and the old man passed away without contempt and insult. [The old man] was Mr. Qin Bowei, one of the most famous T.C.M. practitioners of his generation, and a shining star in the field of contemporary T.C.M.

Master Qin had served as advisor to the State Health Ministry, was a standing member of the academic committee of the Beijing T.C.M. College, and was vice Chairman of the Chinese Medical Association. He was a member of the Pharmacological Committee of the State Science Commission, a member of the Editing Committee of the Pharmacopoia, a member of the Central Committee of the Peasant Worker Democratic Party of China, and a member of the second, third, and fourth National Political Consultative Conference.

Mr. Qin devoted his life to the development of Traditional Chinese Medicine and had [acquired] a profound mastery of the healing arts. He worked his heart out to carry forward the healing arts and to train generations of practitioners to come. His knowledge was expansive and his experience was rich. [Master Qin] was well known for his writing, leaving over sixty books, totaling more than ten million characters. His books ranged from *Highlights of the Medical Practitioners from the Qing Dynasty,* which was written in his early years and consisted of a summary of over twenty famous practitioners of the Qing, to the manuscript *Qiān Zhāi's Medicine,* an exquisite elaboration of T.C.M. theory that he wrote late in life.[1] All his works embraced the theoretical heritage of his predecessors and the initial innovations of the ancient classics. Not only were his theories unique, but they were also of great practical value. He wrote a wide variety of medical essays, historical stories, poems, and verses. Two special columns in the *Health News [Jiàn Kāng Bào]* entitled "Forest of Medicine" and "Chat Following Clinical Practice" were established at his suggestion.

---

[1]Qiān Zhāi was Qin Bowei's scholarly name.

Qin's given name was Zhī Jì. His style name was Bó Wèi and his scholarly name was Qiān Zhāi. He was born in Ché Hēng township in Shanghai County, China on June 6, 1901 of the lunar calendar. Qin was born during midsummer in the southern region of China when the lotus flowers were in full bloom. It is perhaps for this reason that he had a profound love of flowers and he wrote a number of poems praising the lotus, which is "free from any taint even though it grows out of the muck of the swamp." He often reminded us that to be a human being one must have integrity and to be a doctor one must abide by the code of medical ethics. To be in financial poverty reflects nothing more than a lack of internal drive, to be degraded reflects nothing more than a lack of aspiration, and the absence of will never made one a good doctor.

The ninth edition of the *Primer of T.C.M.*, which was written by Master Qin and published in 1981, adopted a simple and elegant lotus flower on the cover page in memory of him. Qin spent his last birthday in 1969 in solitude with his health degenerating. Still it is fortunate that his last photograph taken in Capital Studios on that day has been preserved since then.

The given name of Qin's grandfather was Dí Qiáo, styling himself Nǎi Gē, and taking Yòu Chí as his scholarly name. He was particularly adept at poetry, verse, and the ancient classics. He was a painter and calligrapher by profession and practiced Chinese medicine as an avocation. His practice, however, attracted quite a number of patients and he therefore enjoyed a wide-ranging reputation. Dí Qiáo's works included *Notes of the Nèi Jīng Tú, Manuscripts of Yù Píng Huāi Guǎng,* and *The Medical Notes of Yí Chǔ Yuán.* In Qin's *Highlights of the Medical Practitioners of the Qing Dynasty,* thirty-one case histories in the fourteenth chapter were by his grandfather.

Qin Bowei's father, Xī Qí, and his uncle, Xī Tián, both had a good command of Chinese medical theory and were adept practitioners. Born into such a family, Qin began reading medical books at a very early age. He could recite such primers as the "Three Character Medical Verses," "Verse of the Properties of Medicinal Agents," and "Verse of the Pulses." He was absorbed in literature and read insatiably. Later on he studied in Shanghai Number Three Middle School, and in 1919 entered the Shanghai Medical School established by Dīng Gānrén. Qin proved to be a diligent student, graduating in 1923 as the foremost student of his class.

This [educational background] laid a firm foundation for him to embark on the path of Traditional Chinese Medicine. As one Chinese adage goes, "diligence serves as the path to the mountain [peak] of books and painstaking effort serves as the boat on the infinite ocean of learning." He was renowned for his overall understanding of the T.C.M. literature available at the time, his articulation of the strengths and weaknesses of the different schools of learning and his unique opinions when confronted with confounding arguments. He devoted himself to the study of the *Nèi Jīng* and *Nàn Jīng, Shāng Hán Lùn,* and *Jīn Guì Yào Luè,* often identifying these four books with the "Four Books of Confucius and Mengzi," the *Lùn Yǔ, Mèng Zǐ, Dà Xué,* and *Zhōng Yōng.* He claimed that to be a scholar one could not ignore the "Four Books of Confucius and Mengzi" and to be a Chinese medical practitioner one could not fail to read the *Nèi [Jīng], Nàn*

[Jīng] or the theories of Zhòngjǐng. He felt that one must be deeply rooted in these academic sources and that only by doing so would one avoid becoming a physician who treats the head for a headache and the feet for a pain in the foot.

Master Qin also felt that one must not only be familiar with these medical works and be able to recite them fluently but that a person should take notes while reading these books. One should delight in the accumulation of knowledge, but the manner in which it is acquired should be flexible. Comparison, verification, classification, and enumeration should be emphasized. His *Notes to the Reading of the Nèi Jīng,* published in 1929, were based on many years of voracious reading; [this] is a prime example of this approach.

Even late in life Qin recalled the instructions of the Master Physician Ding Ganren with deep affection. He recalled that when he first became one of Mr. Ding's students, Mr. Ding requested that everyone recite all 220 essays in *Gu Wen Guan Zhi.* Everyone in his class recited one of the essays each day, and such well known masterpieces as *Chū Shī Biǎo* by Zhū Géliàng and *Hòu Chè Bì Fù* by Zhū Shè were memorized thoroughly. The students initially found it boring but as their competence in the classical language improved daily, they ultimately found it much easier to read extensively. For this reason, Master Qin expected us to learn ever more literature and history and to nurture our appreciation of literature. He once said that the single-minded research of Chinese medicine is comparable to the digging of a canal, while the general enhancement of literary appreciation can be likened to the creation of vast rivers and seas.

Famous masters tend to produce extraordinary students and among Qin's classmates were Méng Xuěchéng, Chì Gōngzhāng, Zàn Chéngzhāng, and Wéng Dōngwáng, all of whom have great reputations in the field of contemporary Chinese medicine. Prior to the liberation, Qin, Cheng, and Chi were referred to as the "Three Outstanding [Ones]" of the Shanghai medical community. Cheng was particularly adept in Shang Han theories, while simultaneously being a follower of Yè Guì (Yè Tiānshì). Chì Gōngzhōng was skilled in the application of materia medica. Qin was famous for his mastery of the *Nèi Jèng* and was known in the medical community as "Qin Nèi Jèng."

Qin was well known for his skill in poetry, calligraphy, and medical practice. In his early years he joined the South Club established by Yà Zǐliǔ and was considered the youngest poet of the club.[2] At the age of thirty he published a collection of poems, and by forty had published seven volumes, including supplements to the previous collections, amounting to 344 works. He was a follower of the calligrapher Zhī Qiànzhàng, whose [work] was characterized by its regular style. His characters were brushed smoothly and harmoniously and he only rarely brushed in the casual style. Qin also imitated Mào Wēnyǎng in the ancient style of calligraphy. One parallel poetic sentence that decorates the guard temple of the garden city in Shanghai was a vestige of his early calligraphies. The enormous strength and spirit of the characters were vividly evident in this piece of art work. In actuality his talents reached beyond these fields. He was an

[2]Trans: Yà Zǐliǔ was a well known scholar and social activist who died in the 1960's.

adept draftsman, skilled at drawing plum blossoms, orchids, bamboo, chrysanthemums, and lotus. Qin also loved the exquisite art of carving, sealing, and printing.

Upon graduation, Qin began to practice Chinese medicine, while at the same time teaching in the School of Chinese Medicine. He was elected as secretary of the Chinese Medical Society of Jiang Su Province in 1924.[3] He later founded The New Chinese Medical Club and was Chief Editor of the journal known as *"The World of Chinese Medicine."* In collaboration with Yī Rénwán of Háng Zhōu and Shèng Xuānwáng of Sū Zhōu, he founded the Shanghai College of Traditional Chinese Medicine in 1928, located in Zá Běi District in Shanghai.

Qin undertook the post of instructor himself and devoted himself to research and writing. He would work from morning until night, without a single day of vacation. His approach to teaching was to conduct preliminary theoretical classes on a large scale, distributing assignments and correcting them personally. He would arrange for tutors to help those whose language skills were poor. After three years of study his students began an apprenticeship. He would conduct a nightly discussion session about the clients seen that day and would raise questions, letting the students discuss them. He would also have each student write a case history for the same patient, which he would carefully correct, and these would be circulated among his apprentices. These materials were sometimes edited and compiled. Entitled the "Collection of Qin and his Students," they were exchanged with collections from other localities.

In two decades about five to six thousand students were trained at his school. Textbooks published by the Alumni of Qin['s teaching] in 1930 include physiology, pharmacology, diagnostics, internal medicine, gynecology, and pediatrics. The book called "Practical Chinese Medicine," published by Shanghai T.C.M. Book Bureau, included physiology, pathology, diagnosis, pharmacology, prescription techniques, treatment techniques, internal medicine, gynecology, external medicine, pediatrics, and venereal disease. All these books were based on [Qin's] teaching manuscripts.

In 1930 Qin founded a T.C.M. instruction center in Shanghai, which trained over 1000 participants from all over the country, as well as some overseas Chinese. A monthly journal was published for exchanging academic articles and clinical experience, as well as for answering medical questions. This was actually an unprecedented example of correspondence education in the field of T.C.M., which greatly promoted the popularity of Chinese medicine.

Qin founded a T.C.M. rehabilitation center on Lián Yún Road in Shanghai in 1938. A branch unit was formed in the western part of the city at the same time. Qin Bowei served as superintendent of both the center and the branch unit. This center had over 110 beds and specialized in internal and external medicine, orthopedics, gynecology, and pediatrics. During this time, *"Zhōng Yī Liáo Yǎng Zhuān Kan,"* a special newsletter, was published, which was quite popular with both patients and practitioners.

---

[3]Trans: Shanghai was then one of the cities under the jurisdiction of Jiang Su Province.

Qin often quoted a passage from the classics to describe the relationship between the teaching and learning process. [He would say that] learning makes you aware of your insufficiencies and teaching makes you aware of your frustration. He said that many difficult issues were answered as a result of illuminating questions by fellow students. He [always] insisted on conducting classes [himself] even at an advanced age. In 1961 at the age of sixty he gave our fellow students the same quality of lecture on internal medicine as he always had [when younger], explaining everything thoroughly with the use of simple but thought-provoking examples. His loyalty to the teaching of T.C.M. was vividly displayed.

The Guomintang government held the first central conference on health in 1929, during which a resolution put forward by Yán Yú was adopted, aimed at abolishing Chinese Medicine. The resolution argued that as long as the old medicine remained, the course of modern medicine could not move forward. Subsequently six rules were enacted that included practitioners of Chinese medicine. They were forced to accept "trainings," they were prohibited from the distribution [of medical literature] and from opening medical schools. News of these developments aroused massive indignation and resentment. T.C.M. organizations all over the country elected and sent representatives to Shanghai to oppose this reactionary policy.

On March 17, 1929, a National conference of representatives of Chinese medicine and pharmacology was held in Shanghai and Qin Bowei was elected as the secretary. A petition group was formed following the conference which went to Nán Jīng to demand that the Guomintang government annul the resolution. As a result of the protest of medical practitioners from all over China, and with the massive support of the people, the Guomintang authorities were forced to abolish their resolution. This was a great victory in the struggle of Chinese medicine and was the origin of March 17th as the Chinese medical festival. Qin was always in the vanguard during the struggle, contributing to the struggle to maintain and carrying forward the medical heritage of the motherland.

When giving a talk on the evening of March 16, 1964, in the Affiliated Hospital of Beijing T.C.M. College, Qin described the events of 35 years before with great emotion. Referring to the above incident in a condolence message delivered on September 8, 1978, Fāng Jì said that Qin never yielded and waged a forceful struggle with the dark old society during a time when T.C.M. was reviled and devastated.

Following the liberation, Qin worked as the Chief of the Department of T.C.M. Internal Medicine at No. 11 Hospital in Shanghai. During the winter of 1954 he was personally visited on a number of occasions by Zǐ Huàguō, then the assistant Health Minister, who invited him to be the T.C.M. advisor to the ministry in Beijing. Although reluctant to leave his home town he finally left for Beijing in 1955. He first settled in the dorms of the Health Ministry in the west of Gǔ Lóu in Beijing. When the Beijing College of T.C.M. was formally established in 1956 outside Dōng Zhí Mén in Beijing, for the sake of convenience for teaching and clinical work, Qin moved to live in the simply furnished staff dorm of the T.C.M. college.

Qin set strict demands for himself in the academic field. "Live to learn and learn till senility" was his motto. He often said that academic learning recedes if it is not advanced. When he was an advisor to the Health Ministry in the 1950's, he would study and work until midnight despite having to deal with administrative business. He was a smoker and tended to smoke heavily while contemplating essays and articles, and [he] would often note his initial ideas on the back of a cigarette wrapper. The manuscripts of many of his articles and books were conceived in this way. He once commented jokingly that writing on the back of cigarette wrappers was better than on [file] cards because in addition to being economical they are also less conspicuous. Whenever you have an idea you can write it down, [he said,] regardless of where you are, at a meeting, during a break or while riding in a car. Qin's masterpiece, *Qiān Zhǎi Yī Xué Jián Gáo,* was actually composed of hundreds of manuscripts written on cigarette packages. These unique manuscripts were unfortunately burnt during the cultural revolution.

Qin Bowei had a profound love of Chinese medicine and devoted himself to the healing arts. He would often say that one cannot do good work if one doesn't love and devote oneself to the path one is engaged upon. One can achieve great accomplishments only when one absorbs oneself in what one is doing. He often related holiday and recreational events to medical study and practice and would use common sense to broaden our way of thinking. One mid-summer evening in 1963, a young lady entered the room where we were chatting after dinner. We smelled an aroma of perfume as the lady passed by, waving her sandalwood fan, and commented quietly as we sat around Qin that the smell was immediately nauseating. Qin grinned and said that this was what was called individual preference. You may like the plain palm fan from your home town better than the aromatic sandalwood fan. The T.C.M. treatment of patients should also be based on individual circumstances, specific patterns of symptoms, the localities, and the time of their occurrence. One should not stick to rigid formulas to treat a living person. Furthermore, one should not in the least mimic what others are saying, rather one should consider a problem independently.

He [then] used the example of the treatment of coronary heart disease. [The] medicinals [that] are employed to quicken the blood [and are employed] in removing stasis as well are aromatic medicinals with swiftly wandering functions. He commented that while this is effective from a pharmacological point of view, the individual characteristics of the patient should not be neglected. The following day, Qin took us to #301 hospital for a consultation. The patient was a female over 30 years old who was suffering from coronary heart disease. In looking over the the the case history, the medicinals used by previous doctors included: *dān shēn* (salvia [root], *chuān xiong,* (ligusticum [root])), *chì sháo yào* (red peony [root],) *hú jiāo* (pepper), and *sū mù* (sappan [wood]). However, the patient had vomited the prescription immediately upon taking it. Mr. Qin had been called in five days previously, but had not been able to see her until that day. Qin questioned the patient intensively and when he learned that the sensation of vomiting was induced by the aromatic smell of sandalwood he simply removed this ingredient from the existing prescription.

The following day Master Qin was informed that the patient had not vomited again, that her condition had taken a sharp turn for the better, and that she was in good spirits. Mr. Qin looked pensive and said that we have to learn from what other people have accomplished and not neglect the strong points of other practitioners. In this case the existing therapeutic measures were correct and should be assimilated. At the same time, however, we should pay attention to individual characteristics. This is what is known as understanding the common while attending to the specific. We should never become those mediocre doctors who only feel the pulse with [their] eyes closed and mouth shut tightly, or who deliberately make things complicated to show off. We must seek the truth from fact; the four diagnostic methods of inspection, listening and smelling, inquiry, and palpation should never be neglected, and this is especially true of inquiry.

Master Qin advocated a simultaneous combination of bequeathing and carrying forward Chinese medicine in practical work. He felt that without inheriting [the old wisdom] there could be no development, just as castles in the air are a mirage and so are groundless. He also said that Chinese medicine is not metaphysically confusing, nor is it high-flying and lacking substance, rather it is a pragmatic science. We should proceed from a pragmatic perspective and avoid paying excessive attention to the wording [of the classics].

Master Qin also promoted the cooperation of both Western and Chinese medicine in implementing their benefits and avoiding their shortcomings. He emphasized the scientific patterns of differentiation used in T.C.M. and strongly opposed the idea of simply using herbs and abandoning medical theory.

To give an example of this, one leader of the government suffered from incessant hiccuping. The previous doctor had administered large doses of *mù guāi* (chaenomeles [fruit]), and other medicinals intended to relieve the spasm of the diaphragm. This was not effective and induced acid regurgitation. When Master Qin was called in, his analysis was that the hiccup was probably caused by a spasm of the diaphragm from the Western medical perspective. In Chinese medical treatment, however, the differentiation of symptom patterns is emphasized more than research on specific diseases, formulas, or constituents. This patient was advanced in years and his illness was longstanding. His tongue was red with a little coat and his pulse was thready and weak. This was ascribed to a vacuity of both qi and yin and required vigorous supplementation. Upon inquiry Qin learned that the condition was a result of anger causing a counterflow of qi. If this were the case, medicinals to regulate and descend the flow of qi should have been used. However there was [also] a question as to which specific medicinals should be administered, as there are a wide variety of medicinals that influence the qi. Given the frequent attacks of hiccuping [in association] with a low voice that was due to the failure of the kidney to absorb the qi, the medicinals of choice were those that supplement the kidney and absorb the qi. Master Qin simply prescribed two ingredients, *xī yáng shēn* (American ginseng), and *chén xiāng* (aquilaria [wood]). The first dose relieved the symptom and the second cured it completely.

Premier Zhou [Enlai] was told the story on a subsequent visit to this leader and praised the wonders of Chinese medicine. Master Qin later commented that *Sì Mò Yǐn* [Four Milled Ingredients Beverage] in the ancient formula manual *Jì Shēn Fāng,* conveys the same meaning. Chinese medical treatment is first of all reliant on correct diagnosis, then we must inherit the ancient instructions, while not being limited by the ancient forms. We must think more when we practice Chinese medicine. Mengzi said that if one believes the books one hundred percent then it would be better if there were no books at all. Only in understanding this quotation thoroughly can we achieve what we intend [in the treatment of illness].

During his lifetime, Master Qin was invited to the Soviet Union and Mongolia for medical consultations and academic exchanges. There he primarily treated difficult and complicated cases such as leukemia, hemophilia, and myasthenia gravis and with his treatment he generally achieved the expected effect. He said that we should not be afraid of those conditions considered incurable and [that] they must be dealt with. Needless to say, curing them is not an easy job, but good use should be made of the time while a patient is still alive by increasing their vitality while the condition is stable and controlling the progression [of the illness] when it is volatile. It is therefore possible and pragmatic to minimize the sufferings of the patient and to prolong their life. If we can deal with even a few such cases, it is of extreme benefit to our clinical work. However, we should not bite off more than we can chew, nor should we be to eager for quick success and instant benefit. We must be down-to-earth and accumulate experience. He believed that these incurable conditions will ultimately be finally conquered and that Chinese medicine would discover a way out.

In 1965, at the behest of the leaders of the government, Master Qin underwent an overall medical checkup at Xié Hé Hospital in Beijing. He was deemed to be in good health but when he plunged himself into the task of chronicling his life experiences, he suffered from lobar pneumonia which resulted in fever and hemoptysis. As a result of the drastic change in his life, compounded by the emotional abuses of the tumultuous years [the cultural revolution], he survived the disease [through a celebate lifestyle]. Yet the lack of both restful recuperation and careful medical treatment [contributed to] a more malicious condition [that] began to sprout in the dark.

Eleven years have passed since Master Qin passed away. His teachings, however, are still as fresh as if they happened yesterday. At a time when Spring has returned to the motherland, in keeping with Qin's wishes, we have collected those articles, written between February 1955 through February 1965, that have never been previously published officially as well as those published essays that reflected Master Qin's unique viewpoints and rich experience. Included in this book is also part of Master Qin's personal letters pertaining to Chinese medicine and pharmacology. These articles, essays, and letters have been arranged in chronological order as a token of our profound remembrance.

Da Zhengwu and Feng Qiwang

1981

DISCUSSION OF LIVER ILLNESSES[1]

Definition of Liver Illnesses

There are a great many techniques that are very effective in the treatment of liver illnesses in Chinese medicine. Based upon my personal experience, it is my belief that theory and clinical [experience] are intimately connected. This relationship has a direct bearing on the use of terminology, symptomatology, diagnosis, and treatment, and these aspects in turn influence the prescriptions and medicines that are typically used. This essay is divided into five sections (dealing with the above-mentioned topics). By contrasting these five general discussions, each of which relates to the treatment of liver illness, a dependable basic training will be provided.

1. ON TERMINOLOGICAL IMPLICATIONS IN LIVER ILLNESSES

Our predecessors had a deep understanding of liver illness; however, given the many aspects of terminology, the meaning of some terms is unclear, and there are some cases where what was originally clear has been misunderstood by later generations. For instance, physiological terms are now often confused with pathological terms, and this confusion extends to the names of illnesses as well.

The names of [liver] illnesses vary. They are based on the clinical appearance of pathological changes within the liver viscus,[2] the etiology of the illness, and the nature of the pathological changes observed. What an illness is called also varies with changes in pathology. Beyond this, since pathological changes in the liver viscus may produce symptoms of illness in other viscera, and diseases of other viscera may involve liver symptoms, these conditions are also frequently described as liver illnesses. Thus the distinction between primary and secondary [liver illnesses] becomes blurred and cause and effect are transposed.

---

[1]Qin Bowei is speaking here of liver illnesses as those patterns and disease entities pertaining to the Chinese medical concept of the liver.

[2]In his writing Qin Bowei frequently – and somewhat idiosyncratically – uses expressions such as "liver viscus," a two character expression, one of which is "liver" the second of which is "viscus." This expression emphasizes the distinction between the viscus and the channel.

I believe that before the treatment of liver illnesses can be discussed, the salient concepts pertaining to the terminology used in the discussion of liver illness must be clearly explained. These principles can then be successfully used to guide clinical practice, producing a proper discrimination of patterns and supporting the execution of [effective] treatment. This is the meaning of the adage, "if the titles are correct, the words follow, and if the titles are incorrect, the words will not follow."

Liver Vacuity

This is a physiological term. The liver stores the blood. In general it is said that liver vacuity will be accompanied by many indications of insufficiency of liver blood and in clinical practice the symptoms of liver [qi] vacuity will also often be seen along with symptoms of blood vacuity. The salient symptoms are dizziness, emaciation, a fine pulse, a pale tongue body, and, in women, scanty menses, pale menses, and amenorrhea.

As to liver physiology as a whole, it is said that blood is the substance and that qi is the manifestation; blood is yin and qi is yang. This is referred to as "yin substance and yang function." Symptoms of liver vacuity therefore fit the category of blood depletion and insubstantiality [tǐ bù chōng], as well as the category of debilitation of qi and ineffectuality. These [categories] include qi, blood, yin, and yang and therefore there are four categories [of liver yang vacuity]: vacuity of liver blood, vacuity of liver qi, vacuity of liver yin, and vacuity of liver yang.

We usually say that liver qi and liver yang have an upbearing and smoothing capacity. Thus we have come to refer to this as yòng (function). Illnesses of qi counterflow and hyperactivity of yang are generally referred to as liver qi and liver yang patterns. When [these patterns are] seen [in patients] presenting with lassitude, anxiety, timidity, headache, numbness, and lack of warmth in the extremities, they are called liver qi vacuity and liver yang vacuity patterns. Shèng Huì Fāng states:

> Cold develops in the case of liver vacuity, and with cold there will
> be subcostal distension, chills and fever, abdominal fullness and
> anorexia, depression, paranoia, blurred vision, eyes producing
> black flowers [(i.e., black spots)], bitter taste in the mouth,
> headache, joint problems, contracture of the sinew vessels, brittle
> nails, a tendency to worry and fearfulness, an inability to take a
> deep breath, and a pulse that is deep and slippery. All of these are
> symptoms of liver vacuity.

This vacuity includes both liver blood and liver qi, and it is said that "if there is liver vacuity then cold is engendered."[3] Cold implies an insufficiency of yang. As regards the treatment of liver illnesses this point is extremely important. If these terms are taken [by clinicians] to be merely pathological terms and the sole effort attempted is to understand the pathological context, while ignoring [the liver's] normal physiological function, this is obviously inadequate. Also, in liver vacuity patterns, if one's efforts are directed exclusively at understanding the pathological content

---

[3]Trans: That is, in the case of a pure vacuity of blood and qi there is no pathological heat, and this provides the environment for the production of pathological cold.

while ignoring [the liver's] normal physiological functions, such an approach is obviously flawed.

How can liver qi and liver yang, liver blood and liver yin be distinguished in terms of physiology and pathology? In my experience, liver yang and liver yin form the foundations of liver qi and liver blood. In the practices of our predecessors it was recognized that the qi and blood of the liver viscus are each used by the body in a different manner. Therefore, in regard to liver yang and liver yin, these were differentiated in a manner similar [to that used for the differentiation of] the fire and water of kidney *mìng [mén]*, that is, as kidney yang and kidney yin respectively. Therefore, for the qi and blood of the liver viscus, blood is substance and qi is function or activity. For the liver as a whole viscus, the qi and blood are substance, and yin and yang are activity. Liver yang and liver yin are definitely not abstract terms [applied] outside the context of qi and blood. In fact, neither liver qi nor liver blood may be separated from one another.

Liver Qi

This is a physiological and pathological term as well as a disease name. At present, it is considered to be equally a pathological designation and a disease name describing an excessive strength in the liver viscus that produces pathological symptoms. The form that a liver qi disease assumes is primarily the result of an irritation of the emotions that creates a disharmony of the qi dynamic of the liver viscus. [Thus liver qi disease] appears [clinically] in the form of a horizontal counterflow that may extend further to influence other viscera. The *Lèi Zhèng Zhì Cái* states:

> The nature of liver wood is that of ascension and dissipation, and an obstructive depression[4] [of qi] should not be allowed to develop. If there is depression, the qi of the channels will counterflow, creating eructation, distension, vomiting, sudden anger, costal pain, thoracic fullness, anorexia, early morning diarrhea,[5] and hernia [kuì shān]. All these conditions are symptoms of a horizontal rupture of liver qi.

Its primary symptoms are pain from thoracocostal distension and fullness and lateral abdominal distension and pain.[6] In women, breast distension and pain will also be reported. The outstanding characteristic is distension: pain develops because the qi dynamic becomes distended and static. Therefore, there may be distension and no pain in liver qi illnesses, but there is never pain without distension.

The illness develops first at the location of the [root] viscus and channel. Obviously, this is mainly in the bilateral costal and lateral abdominal regions. [The illness] later diffuses along the channels, upward into the breast and downward into the genital area. It may also influence the spleen and stomach, presenting symptoms of failure to dissipate and transform such as torpid intake, eructation, vomiting, and diarrhea.

---

[4]Trans: Qin Bowei's following discussion of liver depression will clarify this.

[5]Trans: Notice that early morning diarrhea (so-called "cock's crow diarrhea") is a classic symptom of kidney yang vacuity, yet here Qin Bowei also identifies it with liver qi.

[6]Trans: See the discussion of lateral abdominal pain in section two for the details of Qin Bowei's use of this term.

Therefore, these are commonly referred to as symptoms of wood restraining earth. Also, because there is stagnation of the qi dynamic, this stagnation causes the emotions to abruptly counterflow and become inhibited, leading to anger, irritation, and an unsettled spirit.

On the other hand, following an irritation of the spirit, if symptoms of horizontal counterflow of liver qi do not appear and there is instead a depressive binding of liver qi – although both counterflow and binding are illnesses of the qi aspect – rather than calling this liver qi, it is referred to as liver depression. This liver depression will be discussed later. What must be explained here is that liver depression that is not soothed may transform to a liver qi illness. Nevertheless, if a horizontal counterflow of [liver qi] has already occurred, it is impossible for liver qi to transform back to liver depression.

The attack of liver qi on the stomach or its restraint of the spleen may both be explained in terms of wood restraining earth. However, liver depression also influences the spleen-stomach and this condition fits the category of wood not restraining earth. [This situation,] however, cannot be regarded in the same way [as an attack of liver qi]. Regardless of whether it is a illness of liver depression or of liver qi, we must attend to the physiological aspects of the liver qi as well as the regulatory functions of the liver. This attention to liver physiology enables us to avoid excessively coursing or disinhibiting the qi, or eroding and dissipating it in a manner that impairs the proper function of liver qi.

Liver Depression[7]

This is a pathological term as well as the name of an illness. It denotes a failure of orderly reaching and a failure to soothe inhibition within the qi and blood of the liver viscus. In general, the precursors of qi depression may be an initial depressive binding of the emotions that produce depressive qi with an obstructive influence on blood circulation that results in blood depression. If the depression is located in the qi aspect, symptoms such as oppression, unhappiness and despondency, fullness in the thoracocostal region, and poor digestion appear. If the depression is located in the blood aspect, additional symptoms such as intense stabbing costal pain, emaciation of the flesh, and irregular menses appear. Depressive binding of liver qi is generally the exact opposite of liver qi. Liver qi symptoms are effectively those of excessive strength and excessive coursing and draining, and are therefore characterized by horizontal counterflow.[8]

Depressive binding of liver qi [that is not characterized by counterflow] is ineffectual, i.e. there is an inability to course and drain and therefore this condition is characterized by despondency. At the same time, the liver qi [counterflow] pattern is capable of attacking the stomach and restraining the spleen. [This condition is] characterized by symptoms of

---

[7]Trans: Qin Bowei places this discussion after his discussion of liver cold. As the concepts of liver qi and liver depression are so closely related we have rearranged their order for the English edition. Liver heat follows liver fire in the original text.

[8]Trans: In the following sections Qin Bowei provides definitions of "to course" and "to drain," along with other terms.

poor digestion, and thus the liver qi pattern fits the category of an effulgence of wood restraining earth.

Depressive binding of liver qi may also influence the middle burner, manifesting in the spleen/stomach with symptoms of glomus and fullness, which relates to wood not coursing earth. What liver qi and liver depression have in common is that they are both illnesses of the qi aspect, and they both require the use of methods for rectifying and regulating. However, since they each have a different nature, the use of medicinals varies accordingly.

Another characteristic of depressive liver patterns is that because there is a depressive binding of the emotions with worry and anxiety, and the qi dynamic is not soothed, then, over time, this [depressive binding] will transform into heat. This heat is also depressive and deep-lying and is therefore not easily drained. It is characterized by irritation, worry and indignation, yellow and dark urination [and so forth], and is not the same as a surging of liver fire. Depressive heat thus wears the qi, scorches the blood, and over time gradually depletes the body. This is characterized by symptoms of taxation such as tidal fever, night sweats, insomnia, palpitations, and irregular, rough, and slight menstruation in women. Therefore, a synthesis of the entire process of depressive liver symptoms begins with the qi; it progresses to involve the blood, finally consuming [both the qi and blood].

In other words, the depressive liver pattern first arises in the qi aspect and is not as yet a vacuity pattern. As it develops, however, it may influence the blood aspect and become a vacuity pattern. To be sure, during the course of an illness this depressive binding of liver qi is capable of transforming to liver qi, or liver depression, which may in turn generate heat and transform into liver fire. Nonetheless, it should be remembered that liver depression and liver heat will not necessarily transform into liver qi and liver fire. On the other hand, they may already have transformed into liver qi and liver fire. These are two completely different levels and two distinct patterns that must not be confused.

The liver pertains to the category of wood and so liver depression is also called wood depression. Nonetheless, in the *Nèi Jīng* the discussion of wood depression pertains to the category of [illnesses described by] the doctrine of the movement of qi *[yùn qì]* which describes changes in appearance of the natural world. Wood depression is one of the five depressions. The *Yī Guàn* says that the east engenders wood and that fire qi is enclosed therein. If there is wood depression, then earth is depressed. If there is earth depression, then metal is depressed. If there is metal depression, then water is depressed. If there is water depression, then fire is depressed. This is the principle of the mutual engenderment of the five phases and it is understood that if wood is treated, then all the other depressions are cured as well. Also, since the qi is primary in liver depression, it is generally and most frequently qi depression that must be [clinically] considered. Nonetheless, *Dān Xī Xīn Fǎ* states:

> If there is qi depression, then there is depressive damp; and if
> there is depressive damp, then there is depressive heat; if there is
> depressive heat, then there is depressive phlegm; if there is phlegm

depression, then there will be blood depression; if there is blood depression, then there is digestate depression. These are generally indicative of pathological changes and are called the six depressions.[9]

The terms "wood depression" and "qi depression" have different implications. They may be collectively discussed as depressive liver patterns; however, they cannot always be understood as such.[10]

Comparison of Patterns

Pattern	Symptoms
Liver qi depression	Oppression, unhappiness, despondency, thoracocostal fullness
Liver blood depression	the above symptoms, plus stabbing costal pain, emaciation of the flesh, irregular menses.

Translator's Comment

In summary, liver depression is characterized by a general inhibition of liver qi with symptoms of thoracocostal fullness and impaired digestion. There is essentially too much liver qi congested in the liver producing an inhibition of liver qi function throughout the body. If there is also depression in the blood aspect, there will be irregular menses and stabbing costal pain.

Liver qi is characterized by horizontal counterflow with symptoms of thoracocostal pain and distension, including breast distension and pain in women. In this case the liver qi has counterflowed beyond normal liver function and exerts undue influence on other viscera. While there may be a concomitant vacuity of liver blood, according to Qin Bowei the liver blood will only be depressed in the case of liver depression.

While both patterns may negatively influence digestion, liver qi is characterized by the restraining of earth from an effulgence of wood, that is, excessive coursing and draining. Liver depression, on the other hand,

[9]Trans: Qin's point is that while qi depression is the basis of a depressive liver illnesses, the other depressions may easily spring from it.

[10]Wood depression is specific to liver illnesses; however, qi depression is a term for a broader set of illnesses. The six depressions, *liù yù:* qi, blood, damp, fire, phlegm, and food depression. The concept of "free flow" is a key idea particularly in the qi-blood, channel, and triple burner theories. Flow stoppage is thus a major focus of attention in pathology. Depression describes flow stoppage associated with congestion or impairment of flow associated with binding depression. The six depressions, which are the six most typical forms, are readily identifiable:

1. "qi depression," by pain in the chest and lateral costal region, and a deep rough pulse;

2. "damp depression," by general heaviness and pain, or pain in the joints, usually associated with damp weather, and a deep fine pulse;

3. "fire" (or heat) depression," by visual distortion, oppression and restlessness, dark-colored urine, and a deep fast pulse;

4. "phlegm depression," by panting [dyspnea] associated with physical exertion, and a deep slippery pulse;

5. "blood depression," by loss of power in the lower limbs, hemafecia, and a deep scallion-stalk pulse;

6. "food depression," which denotes perduring food, by eructation of sour gas, abdominal distension, and no thought of food and drink.

Of these six, qi depression is the most important, as it underlies all the others; when qi depression is eliminated, the other forms naturally disappear.

characterized by a failure of wood to restrain earth, that is, an inability to course and drain. This has an essential bearing on prescription. Qin Bowei supplies us with a clinical example of this in his discussion of *chái hú* (bupleurum [root]) in section five:

> *Chái hú (bupleurum [root]) upbears and dissipates, and is indicated for depressive stasis of the qi dynamic. However, if a horizontal counterflow of qi already exists, then the use of qīng pí (unripe tangerine peel) and xiāng fù zǐ (cyperus [root]) to course and disinhibit are indicated.*

Both patterns require methods for coursing, draining, and rectifying, however, it is Qin Bowei's assertion that the liver depression pattern requires more coursing and draining, whereas the liver qi pattern requires a greater emphasis on rectification.

Liver depression may produce liver qi. However, according to Qin Bowei liver qi cannot produce liver depression. This is because a lack of circulation is inherent in the definition of liver depression. Imagine a blood blister on your finger; the distension and pain you feel is analogous to that of liver depression. When this blister bursts it will cause its own set of problems of bleeding. This is analogous to the horizontal counterflow that is characteristic of the liver qi pattern.

Liver depression may also produce heat, while strictly speaking, liver qi will not. In speaking of a depressive binding of liver qi, Qin Bowei is referring to the pattern of liver depression. We therefore have liver qi and liver depression which are distinct but related patterns. Depressive binding of liver qi implies liver depression and not liver qi.

Liver Fire

This is a pathological term as well as the name of an illness. When the dynamic of the liver viscus progresses toward hyperactivity – appearing hot in nature and characterized by a surging counterflow – this is called liver fire. The etiology of liver fire is an accumulation of heat in the liver viscus, or the transformation of liver qi into heat. It is said, "If there is a superabundance of qi, there will be fire." Therefore, it is also said, "The presence of qi fire tends toward hyperactivity." Because it is the nature of fire to flare upward, the symptoms most commonly seen are those of headache, unconsciousness, facial heat and facial redness, bitter taste in the mouth, ocular redness, and tinnitus.

An unrestrained surging counterflow may also influence the internal viscera producing a variety of pathological symptoms. The *Lèi Zhèng Zhì Cái* states, "a depression of wood will transform to fire creating symptoms of sour eructation and costal pain, mania, paralysis, reversal, pi, belching, and hemorrhage, all of which are from a surging of liver fire." Clearly these symptoms are produced directly by liver fire, and the manner in which liver fire influences the various internal viscera influences the specific form these symptoms will take. Although the etiology of the illness is that of liver fire, the location of the illness will vary.

Liver fire is sudden and forceful; its clinical presentation is always that of repletion, and in general, it requires direct use of bitter and cold treatment methods. Nevertheless, another aspect [of liver fire] is that fire may injure the yin construction-blood and scorch the fluids; thus it is frequently accompanied by symptoms such as dry throat, binding constipation, and shortened dark urination. Therefore, considering the nature and development of liver fire, we must also pay attention to the aspect of yin vacuity. In recognition of this relationship, our predecessors commonly included medicinals such as *shēng dì huáng* (fresh rehmannia [root]) and *bái sháo yào* (white peony [root]) as assistants in their prescriptions for draining fire.

Liver Heat

This is a pathological term.[11] Liver fire and liver heat have a similar nature; nevertheless, in clinical practice liver heat is indicated by vexation and oppression,[12] dry mouth, heat in the extremities, and dark yellow urine, with no manifestation of surging counterflow. **In my experience, if it is stable, it is heat, whereas, if it moves, it is fire.**[13] Thus the implications of liver heat and liver fire are very different and should also be discriminated by their degrees of intensity.

The etiology of liver heat may be the transformation of an external warm [pathogen]. For instance, the *Nèi Jīng* states:

> In a liver heat illness, the urine first becomes yellow, [then] there is abdominal pain, a tendency to lie down, but an inability to lie calmly, fever, heat contention resulting in manic speech and fright, costal fullness and pain, and agitated limbs.

If external pathogens injure the liver and the qi becomes depressed, transforming to heat, there will be a formation of deep lying heat, or a formation of fire which, when it does not manifest as a surging counterflow, is referred to as depressive heat or depressive fire. Furthermore, because the liver governs the storage of blood, and blood vacuity engenders internal heat, it specifically manifests with symptoms of afternoon tidal fever and a burning fever in the centers of the palms and soles with perspiration. Whenever depressive heat is present in the liver viscus, the construction-blood may also be easily injured. If this situation is left unresolved over too long a time, it will transform into a vacuity pattern.[14]

A transformation of depressive heat may cause vacuity heat and blood vacuity may engender vacuity heat as well. Because the pathomechanisms are not the same, the treatment methods must also differ.

---

[11]Trans: It is not clear why Qin Bowei does not consider liver heat or liver cold illnesses per se. He believes that all the other patterns may be illnesses as well as physiological and/or pathological terms. This may only be a lack of editing in the original Chinese for parallelism but it cannot be assumed that this is the case.

[12]Vexation, *xīn fán:* A feeling of restlessness and irritability that is focused in the heart area is a very common patient complaint that can occur in either vacuity or repletion heat. In severe cases it is associated with agitation, which is increased physical movement.

[13]Trans: Typographical emphasis has been added to this point.

[14]Depressive fire here refers to the intensity of the symptoms, in that depressive fire is more severe than depressive heat. Qin Bowei's differentiation of depressive heat and depressive fire is based solely on the severity of the symptoms, whereas his differentiation of liver fire and liver heat is based on the severity of the symptoms in addition to the presence of movement, a further character of fire that also indicates intensity or severity. The implications of the term "fire" are broad and in context can refer any or all of its aspects.

Liver Yang

This is a physiological and pathological term, as well as the name of an illness. Today, although it is used more often as a pathological term and as the name of an illness, very little consideration is given to its physiological aspects. The term "liver yang" is actually derived from its physiological function. As stated above, the function of the liver viscus has both yin and yang manifestations, and when floating and stirring of the yang is encountered in the clinic, this is called a liver yang symptom.

The etiology of a floating and stirring of liver yang may be either that of liver heat and an ascension of yang, or that of blood vacuity where the yang has not been subdued and stored. The primary symptoms are mental dizziness with slight pain, visual dizziness and photophobia, avoidance of vexation, and an inclination to be quiet. This is also likely to provoke a failure of harmonious gastric downbearing with a presentation of belching, nausea, and vomiting. Nevertheless, in liver yang arising from liver heat there may be also be a simultaneous blood vacuity. When liver yang results from liver blood vacuity, internal heat is very often also present, as the two cannot be separated. In differentiating them, the former [liver heat and an ascension of yang] tends to be a repletion pattern, while the latter [a vacuity of liver blood] is a vacuity pattern.

In general, the nature of liver yang is closely connected with heat and is fundamentally a vacuity pattern. This may be clarified by the recognition that the above statement specifically relates to a vacuity of liver yang presenting as intimidation, headache and numbness, and lack of warmth in the four extremities. Therefore it is said that its nature is intimately related to heat. So is this, or is this a not, a contradiction? It is not. A liver yang pattern also implies a blood vacuity and internal heat with yang rising. **The vacuity here is not in the liver yang itself**. In the event that the liver yang itself becomes diseased, its nature is obviously not the same as this condition. Therefore, clearing, enriching, softening, and calming methods are used in liver yang patterns, so as to subdue and descend; if there is a vacuity within the liver yang itself, warming and nourishing methods must be used to facilitate the liver's capacity for regeneration.

Lín Zhèng Zhǐ Nán Yī Àn points out:

> *Whenever there is a superabundance of liver yang, shells must be used to subdue it, and containment via methods for emolliating and calming are indicated. Sour tastes should be administered to contract it, and they should be assisted by medicinals of a salty descending nature, making sure to clear the heat from the network vessels. Thus it is dissipated and conquered.*

This type of treatment method represents a complete integration of liver yang pathology and also clarifies the intrinsic nature of liver yang itself.

The Nature of Liver Yang

Temperature	Pattern	Repletion/Vacuity	Symptoms
Heat	Stirring of liver yang with an element of blood vacuity	Mixed repletion and vacuity	Dizziness, photophobia, nausea, belching, avoidance of motion, tendency to be quiet
Cold	Vacuity of liver yang	Vacuity	Intimidation, headache, numbness, lack of warmth in the extremities

Liver Yang Treatment

Pattern	Treatment Methods
Mild liver yang	Clear heat, subdue and calm
Severe liver yang	Clear heat, subdue, calm, and nourish the liver

Liver Wind

This is a physiological term as well as the name of an illness. The liver is the viscus of wood and wind. If there is blood vacuity, dryness and wind are generated and this is referred to as liver wind. Because this condition is distinct from external wind and has an endogenous etiology, it is also referred to as "internal wind." It is in the nature of wind to move and shake and its primary symptoms are dizziness to the point of falling down, tinnitus, numbness of the extremities, and twitching. It may give rise to symptoms of nausea and palpitations as well. The *Nèi Jīng* states, "All wind twitching and dizziness pertain to the liver." *Lèi Zhèng Zhì Cái* also states:

> The wind depends upon wood and if there is depression of wood, this transforms to wind, with symptoms of dizziness, vertigo, lingual numbness, tinnitus, spasms, bi, and stroke-like symptoms, all of which are due to the vibratory movement of liver wind.[15]

It also states:

> Liver yang transforms to wind, and upwardly harasses the clear portals resulting in vertex pain, mental dizziness,[16] visual dizziness,[17] tinnitus, palpitations, and vexation causing insomnia [wù fán].

Clinically, all of the above are referred to as liver wind symptoms.

Liver wind and liver yang are two [distinct] symptoms. Liver wind is always due to a transformation of liver yang, thus it is said, "Liver yang transforms to wind," and "Reversal yang transforms to wind."[18] Therefore, wind and yang typically arise together. I believe that liver yang is a pattern associated with internal heat from blood vacuity and a floating of yang. Liver wind appears as a pure vacuity, and may appear not only as

---

[15]Trans: A blood vacuity is implied within the depression of wood referred to here.

[16]Mental dizziness, *yūn:* A subjective whirling sensation, such as is experienced when traveling by ship. Cf. *visual dizziness.* See also the following note.

[17]Visual dizziness, *xuàn:* Clouded flowery vision; often associated with mental dizziness.

[18]See the discussion of liver reversal.

a liver blood vacuity but also as a vacuity of kidney yin. Because of the extreme vacuity of the yin and blood, the liver is unable to moisten and nourish the orifices and the extremities, resulting in the appearance of an incessant vibratory movement. Although this has much in common with liver yang, there are some major practical differences. Clinical evidence indicates that if liver yang is mild, then heat-clearing, subduing, and calming methods are used; if [liver yang] is severe, [however,] these methods are assisted by nourishing the liver.

In the case of liver wind, the liver and kidney must be supplemented, the fluids enriched and the yin nourished. Although calming and draining treatment methods are also used, the methods of using medicinals are different from those used for the treatment of liver yang. In general, when speaking of wind yang, I refer to the presence of the serious symptoms of liver yang. Genuine liver wind however should not be lumped together with liver yang, because, if there is no yang to be subdued, there can be no wind to be extinguished.

Liver Cold

This is a pathological term. Two etiologies give rise to liver cold. The first is a direct penetration of a cold pathogen causing the qi and blood of the liver viscus to congeal. This presents as symptoms of reversal frigidity of the four limbs,[19] abdominal pain, a green-blue-purple hue to the fingernails, a pulse presentation that is fine and wiry or deep, fine, and on the verge of expiry, and the illness will have had a sudden onset. The other condition is a vacuity of yang within the liver viscus itself, with a consequent debilitation of the qi dynamic presenting as lassitude, an inability to endure work, worry, grief, and timidity, chilled extremities, and a pulse that appears deep, fine, and slow. This condition most often has a gradual onset.

Patterns of Liver Cold

Pattern	Vacuity/ Repletion	Symptoms	Pulse	Treatment Methods
Cold pathogens congest the liver	Repletion	Reversal chill abdominal pain, green-blue fingernails	Wiry, deep, fine, on the verge of the expiry	Use acrid and warm medicinals to free yang
Vacuity of liver yang	Vacuity	Lassitude, inability to work, grief and timidity	Deep, fine, and slow	Supplement the root, warm and nourish

As to a yang vacuity of the liver viscus itself, this condition reflects the physiological aspect of an insufficiency of liver yang, presenting as a debility of its dynamic capacity, and so pertains to the category of vacuity cold. In treating vacuity cold, warming and nourishing medicinals should be included to promote supplementation of the root. This [approach] differs from the treatment of a contraction of pathogenic cold where medicinals

---

[19]Reversal frigidity of the limbs, *sì zhī jué lěng:* Severe cold in the limbs associated with desertion, and so forth. Synonym: counterflow frigidity of the limbs.

that are acrid and warm and that free the yang are employed. The essential nature of liver yang has already been discussed several times and if, for instance, one becomes confused deciding between a vacuity of liver yang and a contraction of cold by the liver, there will be a negative influence on the therapeutic effect.

Liver Reversal

This is the name of an illness. Reversal has three meanings; the first is that the qi that should naturally descend instead counterflows upward. The second is counterflow chill of the hands and feet. The third is clouding collapse and unconsciousness. In general, liver reversal is not limited to a single pattern; it includes, however, only the three presentations mentioned above.

If anger and indignation give rise to qi reversal, the symptoms will be those of a sudden clouding collapse, clenched jaws, lack of warmth in the hands and feet, and symptoms that resemble wind stroke.

An ascending attack of liver yang gives rise to clouding reversal[20] with symptoms of active movement of the head and eyes, clouding, collapse and unconsciousness, perspiration, facial pallor, and chilled extremities.

A surging ascension of liver fire gives rise to sudden reversal *[bó jué]* with symptoms of sudden collapse and facial redness, inhibited bronchials, phlegmatic respiration, and a pulse that appears wiry and rapid.

A vacuity of liver and kidney yin with internal wind will give rise to tetanic reversal with symptoms of clouding of the spirit, wooden tongue, vexation, irritation, twitching and spasms in the hands and feet, and a frequent tendency to desertion.[21] These are referred to clinically as liver reversal.

Zhōng Guó Yī Xué Dà Cí Diǎn explains liver reversal as "pathogenic liver distension with intense heat and reversal." This text recognizes the predominant etiology as a simple yin vacuity with an effulgence of fire, from emotional irritation, anger, and unexpected personal loss. These events easily lead to reversal chill of the four limbs, nausea and vomiting, clouding dizziness, epilepsy, and unconsciousness. Treatment with methods for calming the spirit, extinguishing wind, coursing the liver, and resolving depression are indicated.

Unfortunately, once the various types of liver reversal symptoms are mixed together, they become rather difficult to distinguish and are thus ambiguous.

---

[20]Clouding reversal, *hūn jué:* [*hūn,* clouded, hazy; *jué,* invert, turn around]. Sudden loss of consciousness, sometimes accompanied by reversal frigidity of the limbs. It differs from clouding of the spirit in that it is of short duration.

[21]Desertion, *tuō:* [*tuō,* shed, cast off]. Critical depletion of yin, yang, qi, or blood, primarily characterized by pearly sweat, reversal frigidity of the limbs, gaping mouth and closed eyes, limp open hands, enuresis, prolapse of the anus, and a fine pulse verging on expiry. Note: *tuō* means to shed, as a snake sheds its skin. The term is rendered as "desertion" to emphasize the unfavorable associations implied in the medical context because "shedding" in English carries generally more positive associations.

Patterns of Liver Reversal	
Pattern	**Symptoms**
General reversal	Counterflow of qi
	Chill of hands and feet
	Clouding collapse
Qi reversal	Clouding collapse
	Clenched jaws
	Cold hands and feet
	Windstrike
Liver yang reversal	Movement of head and eyes
clouding reversal	Collapse
	Unconsciousness
	Facial pallor
Liver fire	Sudden collapse
sudden reversal	Facial redness
	Bronchial congestion
	Phlegmatic respiration
	Wiry rapid pulse
Vacuity of liver and kidney yin	Clouding spirit
tetanic reversal	Vexation
liver reversal	Irritation and desertion
	Twitching spasms of hands and feet

Liver Repletion

This is a pathological term. When there is liver cold, liver heat, or liver qi not pertaining to vacuity patterns, this is referred to as liver repletion. It states in the *Nèi Jīng,* "If there is a repletion of liver qi, there will be anger." It also states, "If there is liver repletion, then there will be bilateral subcostal pain radiating to the lateral abdominal region and a tendency to anger." The etiology of liver repletion has been clearly described and this idea should not be overgeneralized.

Liver Accumulation

This is the name of an illness and is one of the accumulations of the five viscera. It indicates an enlargement of the liver viscus that [the practitioner] can be feel on palpation. The *Nàn Jīng* states:

> Accumulation of the liver is called fat qi [féi qì]. It is located in the left subcostal region where it has a beginning and is well defined. If left uncured over a period of time, it will cause counterflow cough and kē nuè, persisting for years.

All later discussions of liver accumulation throughout history have been based upon this treatise.

The *Nàn Jīng* also states:

> Splenic accumulation is called pǐ qì [glomus qi] and is located in the chest cavity. The abdomen is large like a boat, and, if left uncured, this will cause loss of use of the limbs, jaundice, and failure of food and drink to transform to flesh.

It is my belief that these two words, "liver" and "spleen," should be reversed so that hepatic accumulations are called *pǐ qì* (glomus qi), and splenic accumulations are called *féi qì* (fat qi). Reversing these terms not only only corrects the [discrepancy in anatomical] locations, but [also provides consistency] in naming these concepts.

Liver accumulation is a result of the initial presence of qi stasis and qi that is not soothed, and is therefore called "glomus qi." Extreme swelling and enlargement of the spleen viscus is therefore called "fat qi," and this is appropriate as well. The specific symptoms of this pattern are hepatic swelling and enlargement with a general feeling of fatigue and taxation, a deep discomfort in the hands and feet, diminished appetite, and emaciation. If left uncured too long, this pattern will often engender symptoms of jaundice and drum distension.[22]

Splenic swelling and enlargement pertains to malarial lump glomus,[23] which commonly causes fatigue taxation giving rise to fever and chills. I suspect this mistake has been perpetuated in the classical literature and so have presented my own views here for discussion.

Liver Fixity [Gān Zhuó]

This is the name of an illness. We see in *Jīn Guì Yào Luè:*

> [In cases of] liver fixity, people typically want to beat their breasts, and from beginning to end during the affliction, yet they still desire hot drinks. Xuán Fù Huā Tāng [Inula Decoction] treats it.

These are symptoms of depressive stagnation of the qi and blood of the liver viscus which fail to circulate. Therefore, treatment methods for downbearing the qi, dissipating bondage, quickening the blood, and freeing the network vessels are employed. Nevertheless, if liver symptoms are not evident, then this cannot be diagnosed as a liver illness because to do so, there must be simultaneous pi fullness, distension, and pain in the costal region. This may also be initially due to liver cold qi stasis that tires the son, resulting in a devitalization of heart yang that in turn has an inhibiting influence on the lung qi. This is why taking hot fluids will diminish the symptoms only at the outset of the illness. At this later stage only heavy emolliating prescriptions will effectivly suppress [depressive stagnation].

The prescription [*Xuán Fù Huā Tāng* (Inula Decoction)] contains *xuán fù huā* (inula flower) and stalks of *xiè bái* (Chinese chive [bulb]), which are

---

[22]Drum distension, *gǔ:* Severe abdominal swelling with a withered yellow coloration of the skin, and prominent green-blue vessels (caput medusae). Causes include damage to the liver and spleen when emotional depression gives rise to disruption of qi dynamic; damage to stomach and spleen due to intemperate eating and alcohol consumption; damage to liver and spleen when qi and blood flow is disrupted in parasite accumulation patterns and other infectious diseases. Drum distension is the result of stagnation and accumulation of qi, blood, and water turbidity in the abdomen, from interrelated illnesses of the liver, spleen, and kidney.

[23]Lump glomus, *pǐ kuài:* A generic term that includes all palpable abdominal masses, which in biomedicine are explained as enlargement of the viscera or the presence of tumors. These are classified in ancient literature as concretions, conglomerations, accumulations, and gatherings. These are sometimes given more specific names such as elusive and bowstring masses, or deep-lying beams. The presence of lump glomi invariably heralds pronounced abdominal distension.

of primary importance for freeing the yang in the upper burner, quickening the blood, and normalizing the qi. My preliminary experiences are advanced here to promote discussion.

Patterns of Liver Fixity

Depressive stasis of qi and blood

Stage	Symptoms	Treatment Methods
Initial	Beating of the breast and desire for hot drinks	Downbear the qi Dissipate bondage Quicken the blood Free the network vessels
Later	Above symptoms plus pi fullness and costal pain	Emolliation

Liver distension, liver water, liver impediment, liver nuè

These are all names of illnesses. They are scattered throughout the *Nèi Jīng* and *Jīn Guì Yào Luè,* and relate to cough, distension fullness, water swelling, impediment pain, and malarial symptoms that simultaneously manifest with liver channel symptoms.

It was the habit of our ancestors to classify symptoms according to the viscera and bowels [with which they were associated]. Thus, in both pathology and treatment the main illness and the main viscus affected were of primary concern. The [illnesses discussed in this section] should not be mistaken for liver illnesses per se. For instance, cough is a symptom of a lung illness, and if [these symptoms are] seen with costal pain or costal distension and fullness, the condition is referred to as a liver cough. The treatment of the lung and the suppression of the cough are of primary importance, assisted by regulation of the liver.

The symptom of liver distension is related to distension and fullness and is seen simultaneously with costal fullness and pain that radiates to the lateral abdominal region.

The symptom of liver water relates to water swelling that is seen simultaneously with subcostal and abdominal pain, making it difficult to turn on one's side.

Liver impediment is related to impediment pain and is seen simultaneously with insomnia and fright vigilance.

The symptom of liver *nuè* is acute malaria seen with a pallid complexion and sighing. In later ages the idea of epileptic patterns developed in which these symptoms were seen in conjunction with green-blue lips and facial complexion, and gan accumulation syndromes presenting with green-blue veins and brain fever [encephalitis]. Such liver symptoms are referred to as being in the category of liver epilepsy or liver gan, although the meaning of the two terms is identical.

The above terms relate to liver illnesses, some of which are physiological and some pathological. Some are also terms for specific illnesses and reflect differences in the primary and secondary stages of a given illness. It is my belief that we must be more rigorously discriminating in the treatment of liver illnesses and that this discrimination can never be ambiguous. At the same time we have a responsibility to rearrange this material for unified understanding.

2. UNDERSTANDING THE PRIMARY SYMPTOMS AND PRIMARY DIAGNOSTIC METHODS IN LIVER ILLNESSES

To diagnose a liver illness we must understand the primary symptoms involved and, at the same time, we must grasp the focal points of diagnosis. Given the relationships between the viscera, liver illnesses will be encountered that do not have an entirely hepatic symptom pattern. The salient symptom pattern, however, will be hepatic. Sometimes in complex symptom presentations [it is largely] the main symptoms that will determine [the treatment approach].

Diagnostic methods generally consist of the four examinations and the eight parameters. However, there are also modalities specific [to liver illnesses], and it is these specific diagnostic points upon which we frequently depend [in clinical practice]. Naturally, one might take a one-sided viewpoint regarding the liver viscera and consequently fail to study it in the context of all the internal viscera. If we suppose that an understanding of the primary symptoms and the salient diagnostic methods relating to liver illnesses by themselves truly enable proper treatment of a liver illness, we are making a fundamental error.

Costal Pain

Costal pain is a common symptom in liver illnesses. A great many illnesses rely upon the presence of costal pain to be diagnosed as a liver illness or to confirm a relationship to the liver viscus. Since the liver channel envelops the ribs, whenever there is injury to the liver from an external pathogen or the seven affects, then there is qi stasis and congelation that may give rise to costal pain. Therefore *Gŭ Jīn Yī Jiàn* states, "Costal pain is an illness of the jue yin liver channel." However, costal pain is not always due to a liver illness, as wind cold and phlegm rheum may also cause its appearance. Nevertheless, it is primarily seen in liver illnesses.

In liver illnesses the appearance of costal pain is due primarily to liver depression, which is itself typically a result of repressed emotion, indecision, or longstanding anger preventing an orderly reaching of liver qi and thus producing an obstruction of the network vessels. The onset of pain and soreness is preceded by distension and fullness with an intermittent pain that gradually increases in intensity. In general, therapy need not go beyond coursing the liver and rectifying the qi. If there is longstanding pain, this will influence the blood aspect. Since blood follows qi, [blood] stasis will develop with symptoms of stabbing pain, or a hot burning sensation. The rectification of the middle should therefore be assisted by methods for quickening and clearing the blood.

In general, costal pain is most often a repletion pattern and is only rarely a vacuity pattern. If there has been a habitual depression of the qi and blood, or if there has been an excessive use of acrid drying medicinals for rectifying the qi, then repletion may transform to vacuity, with symptoms such as continuous indistinct pain, a tendency to fatigue taxation, cephalic dizziness, and visual dizziness. Most often, methods that nourish and harmonize the blood are indicated, assisted by those that regulate the qi.

Regardless of whether costal pain in liver illnesses presents itself within the context of a repletion or a vacuity pattern, it will quite easily produce spleen/stomach symptoms such as diminished appetite, aversion to oily slimy foods, nausea and abdominal distension, and frequent belching. This is a result of an effulgence of wood restraining earth in the case of repletion, and of wood not coursing earth in the case of vacuity. Both conditions influence digestive function. In the latter situation [i.e., wood not coursing earth] the spleen/stomach must be considered [as a focus for treatment], otherwise the greater the accumulation of earth qi, the more the orderly reaching of liver qi is impeded. Although the primary symptoms are in the liver, the harmonizing of the middle and the transformation of dampness take precedence, particularly if the spleen fails to transform dampness and there is an internal hindrance of turbid damp with a thick slimy tongue coat.

Patterns of Costal Pain

Pattern	Symptom	Treatment Methods
Liver depression	Costal pain and soreness	Course the liver and rectify qi
Liver depression and blood stasis	Stabbing pain and burning sensation	Course the liver and rectify qi Quicken and clear the blood
Liver depression and blood vacuity	Continuous indistinct pain and fatigue	Nourish and harmonize assisted by regulation of the qi
Liver depression influencing the stomach and spleen	*See following table*	*See following table*

Differentiation of Liver Depression
Influencing the Stomach and Spleen in Costal Pain

Repletion Pattern	Symptom	Treatment
Wood restraining Earth	Diminished appetite aversion to oily greasy foods Abdominal distension Belching	Course the liver and harmonize the middle (emphasis on the liver)

Vacuity Pattern	Symptom	Treatment
Wood not restraining Earth	Above symptoms plus a thick tongue coat	Harmonize the middle and transform dampness (emphasis on the spleen)

Costal Distension

Subcostal fullness and oppression that is not soothed is a specific symptom of stagnation of liver qi. This [condition] presents itself as a relatively heavy sensation in the chest and diaphragm, or a sense of distension radiating downward into the abdomen. In general this pertains to the category of repletion patterns and is a precursor to costal pain. Therapy therefore also consists of methods for coursing the qi, and thus differs from costal pain only in its degree of intensity.

Lateral Abdominal Pain (*Shào Fù Tòng*)

Lateral abdominal pain pertains to the liver channel. Qi blockage, stasis, and congelation may all cause soreness and pain and are all commonly involved in causing costal pain. In the *Nèi Jīng*, it states:

> *In illnesses of the liver, there will be bilateral subcostal pain radiating to the shào fù [lateral abdominal region] and a tendency to irritability/anger.*

There will be a great deal of pain and simultaneous distension with blood stasis and congelation, [all] as a result of qi blockage. There will be an arresting, urgent, twisting pain [that radiates to the lateral abdominal region] but the treatment method is the same as that used for the treatment of costal pain. This condition is frequently seen in the practice of gynecology. In "dysmenorrhea," premenstrual abdominal pain will be present with [simultaneous] lateral abdominal pain and distension. In extreme situations this condition also involves the costal region. There may be breast distension and pain as well. Treatment is primarily aimed at coursing the liver.

In addition, regarding the location [of the *shào fù,*] it should be pointed out that there is one opinion that it is the area found on either side of the umbilicus, and another opinion that it is the area below the umbilicus. It is also generally understood that ⼩ *shào [fù]* and ⼩ *xiǎo [fù]* are rarely distinguished. This is explained in *Zhōng Guó Yī Xué Dà Cí Diǎn*, which defines *shào fù* [as meaning] "*xiǎo fù.*" It [furthermore asserts that] *shào fù* refers to "the subumbilical area, while the area proximate to the bladder is called the lower abdomen *[xiǎo fù].*" I take this to mean that "*shào fù*" relates to the areas lateral to the umbilicus while *xiǎo fù* relates to the subumbilical area. The *Nèi Jīng* clearly points out that "*shào* connects to the hypochondriac region and radiates into the *shào fù* with pain and distension.*" It also points out:

> *In the case of liver illnesses with mental and visual dizziness and costal fullness, there will be pain in the lumbar spine and lateral abdominal region in three days.*

It is easy to understand then that in these statements the *shào fù*[24] is indicative of the periumbilical area and not the subumbilical area. This has relevance in the diagnosis of liver illnesses and should be thoroughly understood.

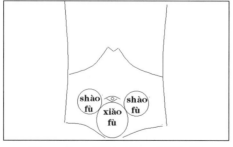

Illustration of Shào Fù and Xiǎo Fù

[24]Trans: The quotation marks around *shào fù* have been added to emphasize that Qin is discussing the term. *Shào fù* is from here forward translated as lateral abdominal pain, while *xiǎo fù* is translated as lower abdominal pain, as this accurately reflects Qin Bowei's use of the terms in Chinese.

Abdominal Distension

Abdominal distension in liver illnesses also tends to be located in the periumbilical area. Sometimes it may be mild and sometimes intense, and is often seen in liver qi patterns. For instance, in examining liver illnesses characterized by abdominal fullness and distension, there is often a concurrent [clinical presentation of] intestinal and gastric symptoms such as extreme postprandial distension and borborygmus that is distinctively relieved by flatulence. Only the abdominal area is enlarged and is drum-like upon palpation. There is a gradual accumulation of water, the skin of the abdomen is strained, the veins are exposed, and it is hard and full upon palpation. This pertains to the category of "simple abdominal distension," and is also referred to as "drum distension."

This condition is most commonly from repressed emotions, immoderate consumption of food and alcohol, and the development of an elusive mass scattered over a large area, which is essentially a congelation of qi and blood of the liver viscus, transforming to involve the spleen.[25] There is an accumulation of qi with water stoppage and therefore, in general, methods for coursing the liver and supplementing the spleen are used. Because there is a liver stasis and hindrance from spleen qi dampness, our predecessors believed that supplementation was contraindicated because it caused a binding accumulation of qi. Warming is contraindicated because it causes wearing injury of the yin fluids. Precipitation is contraindicated because purging promotes a rapid vacuity of the correct qi and tends to create more difficulties in later stages of therapy.

Dizziness

Mental and visual dizziness may either be symptoms of insufficient liver blood, liver yang, or an ascending harassment of liver wind. There may also be a tendency toward severe liver heat that causes an ascending harassment of liver yang with distending pain at the *tài yáng* points (at the temples). Whenever we treat these patterns we cannot deviate from the principles of nourishing the blood, subduing the yang, and clearing heat. Moreover, blood nourishing medicinals that are softening and moistening must be chosen or else there will be a stirring of wind yang. It is also important that we enrich the kidney and foster the yin.

Convulsive Spasm

This is a symptom of liver wind that is due to an extreme depletion of the yin and blood rendering them unable to moisten and nourish the sinew channels. There is therefore acute hypertonicity of the hands and feet with continuous fluctuations in tension. At the onset, wriggling of the fingers may be observed and when the convulsive spasm is serious, it becomes tetanic reversal.[26]

---

[25]Trans: Distension is either the result of accumulation or a physical mass. The mass is due to a congelation of qi and blood in the liver, which influences the spleen. This may be from emotional repression and immoderate dietary intake.

[26]Trans: Wriggling fingers is a mild case of convulsive spasm, while tetanic reversal is a serious case of the same phenomena.

Bitter Taste in the Mouth

Liver heat and gallbladder fluids (i.e. bile) drain externally and this is typically seen in association with a dry mouth. Nonetheless, if there is heat in the gallbladder, this symptom may also appear; therefore, if [this symptom appears] in the absence of [other] liver symptoms, the gallbladder should be treated.[27]

Irascibility

Unrestrained emotional irritation and irascibility are frequently seen in liver qi and liver fire patterns. The *Nèi Jīng* says: "The determination of the liver creates irascibility." It also says: "If there is a repletion of liver qi then there will be irascibility." The etiology of this [condition] lies in the orderly reaching capacity of the liver, which becomes depressed and results in a surging of qi. This surging results in horizontal counterflow, and the horizontal counterflow results in a loss of harmonious disinhibition.[28] Thus the liver tends toward anger. On the other hand, excessive anger injures the liver, and often they have a mutual effect on one another.[29]

Plum Pit Qi

[In plum pit qi] there is a sensation of something being lodged in the throat, although there is no physically apparent foreign object lodged there. The patient cannot swallow it, nor can they spit it up, although it does not hinder eating. Otherwise it may be seen with simultaneous thoracic oppression and shortness of breath, and in these cases is called plum seed qi. This condition is most often due to failure of the liver qi to be soothed, [which in turn] influences the stomach qi, causing qi stasis and congealing phlegm. The patient is unconscious of its development. Aromatic [medicinals] for opening depression are indicated and the liver and stomach should be treated concomitantly.

Shàn Qì

The liver vessel encircles the lower yin, and there is a distending pain and a downward pulling sensation in the testicles that is referred to as *shàn qì*. This is typically because of qi stasis. Zhāng Jǐngyuè said: "In treating shàn, one must first treat the qì," meaning that the liver qi must be coursed and the qi disinhibited. Nonetheless, if cold is involved [in the genesis of a *shàn qì*], the scrotum is not warm; if there is heat [in the genesis

[27]Trans: If the bitter taste in the mouth is from heat in the gallbladder channel, then treat the gallbladder. Symptoms that pertain specifically to the gallbladder include fever and chills, headache, pain in the eye or jaw, subaxillary swelling, and pain along the channel in the hip, leg, or foot. The presence of these symptoms within the context of an overall heat pattern and in conjunction with a bitter taste in the mouth would indicate heat in the gallbladder channel.

[28]Trans: Factors such as dietary immoderation and stress may depress the liver and cause the liver qi to surge beyond its normal bounds. This precipitates a horizontal counterflow of qi resulting in anger and irascibility.

[29]Surging of qi is the name of a pattern of illness first discussed in the *Jīn Guì Yào Luè*. In that context, it is defined as an ascending counterflow of the qi of the *chōng mài* resulting from the presence of deep lying internal rheum pathogens and a vacuity of kidney yang. Its use here in the context of liver qi, however, is synonymous with any violent counterflow of liver qi.

of a *shàn qì*], the urine is shortened and dark; if there is dampness [in the genesis of a *shàn qì*], there is swelling, heaviness, and numbness; in the case of an insufficiency of middle qi, excessive walking, standing, and exertion will aggravate it.

Scrotal Retraction

This is the manifestation of the exhaustion and severance of the essential qi of the liver viscus and is typically seen together with lingual rolling. Because the liver vessel descends and surrounds the genitals, and a network vessel ascends to the base of the tongue, if there is a severance of essential qi of the channels[30] and network vessels, contracture [of the scrotum] and hypertonicity [of the tongue will] result.

Jaundice

In general, this is primarily from dampness and heat of the spleen and stomach as well as from cold damp, so jaundice does not fall within the scope of liver illnesses. Nonetheless, it commonly appears along with liver illnesses. Of note in *Yǔ Yì Cǎo* is the statement:

> Heat in the gallbladder makes the sap full and overflow outward, gradually seeping into the channels and vessels, and making the body and eyes yellow. This is an alcoholic jaundice illness.

The *Lín Zhèng Zhǐ Nán Yī Àn* also states:

> In the development of yang jaundice, dampness is a result of the transformation of fire and internal stagnant heat. The gallbladder heats up and the [bilious] fluid drains, and together with the turbid qi in the stomach, does not pass upward nor is it drained below. This produces a steaming obstructive depression that injures the lung, rendering the body and eyes yellow. Heat flows into the bladder, so the color of the urine becomes dark and yellow like the color of the skin of the red tangerine pit. Yang is bright and treatment lies in the stomach. In the development of yin jaundice, dampness arises from cold water, spleen yang is unable to transform dampness, and the gallbladder fluids are hindered by damp. This soaks the spleen, saturating the flesh and spilling over into the skin and muscle with a blackish yellow color. Yin is dark and treatment lies in the spleen.

This describes the presentation of jaundice relative to the bile. Our ancestors used the principle of miso [production] to explain jaundice, though this is a rather fanciful [analogy]. The gallbladder and the liver have an internal-external relationship and pathological changes within the liver viscus greatly influence the gallbladder, so the presentation of jaundice in liver illnesses is also quite natural.

Jaundice patterns are all characterized by obstruction of damp turbidity, a lack of motility of the stomach and spleen, thick slimy tongue coat, impaired digestion, vomiting, and scanty shortened urination. In

---

[30]Trans: Essential qi is that aspect of the essence that acts to maintain functional activity in the viscera. Essential qi includes both defensive and constructive qi, as well as the acquired essence associated with the kidney. In this case, the essential qi has become disconnected specifically from the liver channel. The resulting loss of nourishment creates scrotal retraction and hypertonicity of the tongue.

general, methods for clearing and transforming, or warming and transforming, and disinhibiting dampness are employed. There are a large number of established prescriptions that treat the liver and gallbladder [in jaundice], such as *Gǔ Dǎn Wán* (Dietary Irregularity Jaundice Pills), which uses *lóng dǎn* (gentian [root]) and *niú huáng* (bovine bezoar); *Yī Qíng Yǐn* (Single Cleaning Drink) which uses *chái hú* (bupleurum [root]) and *chuān xiōng* (ligusticum [root]), or *dāng guī* (tangkuei) and *Qín Jiāo Sǎn* (Large-Leaved Gentian Powder), which uses [medicinals such as *dāng guī* (tangkuei), *chuān xiōng* (ligusticum [root]), and *bái sháo yào* (white peony [root]). Also, when the liver and spleen give rise to drum distension, this will, in severe conditions, also present as jaundice. The yellow color may not be obvious, but there will be a soot black hue especially in the facial area. Methods for disinhibiting damp are in general not sufficient by themselves and must be assisted with selected medicinals from the blood nourishing and harmonizing categories.

Wiry Pulse

A wiry pulse is the predominant [pulse] of the liver viscera; whether it is a healthy pulse, an ill pulse or a death pulse is a question that must be discerned. The presence of liver illnesses should not be determined simply by observing a wiry pulse, and the relative severity of any given liver illness must also be determined [by a complete evaluation].

The primary characteristic of a wiry pulse is its forcefulness, especially the presence of a sharp sensation felt when the practitioner's finger touches the pulse wave. It will be like the sensation felt when touching a steel wire, definitely not soft. Occasionally this pulse may be seen together with a slippery pulse. In this case it is principally a slippery pulse, the wiry sensation under the fingers is sharp and forceful, arriving at the end [of the pulse wave]. This is similar to the tense pulse.

The tense pulse has strength and elasticity, like pressing on a rope but has no sharpness, and this is a significant distinction. In serious stages of liver illnesses, the pulse may appear to be simultaneously tense and wiry with an especially hard rhythm in the cubit, bar, and foot positions, moving straight up and straight down. If it lacks strength on heavy pressure, it is called a drumskin pulse; or if it is deep and not floating, it is called a confined pulse.

In using the wiry pulse to diagnose liver illnesses, we must pay attention to the entire pulse. For instance, if it is wiry and fine, this indicates liver blood vacuity; wiry and slow indicates liver cold; wiry and rapid indicates liver heat; wiry, fine, and rapid is indicative of liver vacuity with internal heat; and wiry, large, and rapid indicates an exuberant effulgence of liver fire. We must also attend to the individual pulse positions. For instance, the left bar pulse is the liver, and liver illnesses in general will most often have a wiry pulse at the left bar position. If the left cubit is wiry, slippery, and rapid, this indicates liver fire causing a stirring of heart fire, which is typically accompanied by symptoms of cardiac vexation and insomnia. If only the right bar is wiry, pathogenic wood restrains earth, which is typically accompanied by symptoms of abdominal pain and diarrhea. Furthermore, when a liver illness produces abdominal fullness, distension, and enlargement, all the pulses on both hands may be wiry, or the right hand pulse may be more exuberant than the left. The illness may then enter a more confused phase where the pulse becomes floating, large, wiry, tense, and rapid, with the cubit more exuberant than the foot, and it will lack strength on heavy pressure.

Also, wiry pulses do not always indicate liver illnesses, nor do liver illnesses invariably have wiry pulses. It is very important to remember that even when a wiry pulse is detected, a discrimination of patterns is still required.[31]

Types of Wiry Pulses

Pulse	Subcategory	Description
Wiry		Feels like a steel wire
Wiry	Slippery wiry	Slippery but forceful at the end
Tense		Strong and elastic but lacking sharpness
Drumskin		Tense but lacks strength on heavy pressure
Confined		Tense and deep, not floating

Wiry Pulses and Patterns

Pulse Pattern	
Wiry and fine	Liver blood vacuity
Wiry and slow	Liver cold
Wiry and rapid	Liver heat
Wiry, fine, and rapid	Liver vacuity with internal heat
Wiry, large, and rapid	Effulgence of liver fire
Wiry at left bar position	Liver illnesses in general
Wiry, slippery, and girdling at left cubit position	Liver fire causing a stirring of heart fire
Right bar wiry	Wood restrains earth
Bilaterally wiry or right more exuberant than left	Abdominal distension and enlargement

Tongue

Tongue sides red, thorny, and green-blue purple

[When] the sides of the tongue are red, thorny, and green-blue purple, there are pathogenic changes in the liver viscus. This is obvious when examining both sides of the tongue. If the [sides] are red there is liver heat, if the [sides] are red and thorny there is liver fire. If they also assume a green-blue purple color like the tips of needles, or form maculae, there is internal blood stasis, which will most often be seen with costal distension and stabbing pain, and so forth.

[31]Trans: Readers who are familiar with the pulse may find these descriptions unsatisfactory. Qin Bowei's point is that a slippery wiry pulse is basically a slippery pulse. His description here emphasizes the wiry quality as a means of bringing his idea into focus. Regarding the relationship between a pulse that is wiry and slippery at the left cubit position, notice that while we commonly associate slippery pulses with either phlegm, pregnancy, or profound good health, a slippery pulse may also be indicative of heat.

Tongue body hard or soft, retracted or tremulous

Tongue bodies that are rigid, move uncontrollably, are shortened, retracted, flaccid and soft, stretched, tremulous, or deviated all indicate liver wind.

Tongue Patterns Pertaining to the Liver	
Tongue	**Pattern**
Red sides	Liver heat
Red and thorny sides	Liver fire
Green-blue purple sides with maculae	Internal blood stasis

Green-blue complexion

Green-blue is the color of the liver and patients who suffer from long-standing liver illnesses often have a green-blue hue or a somber yellow color, with a predominantly dark cast on the forehead. Children suffering from acute fright wind[32] often have a green-blue [facial] color and green-blue veins on their face from the arousal of liver heat; or, if there is long-standing wind fright from liver effulgence and spleen weakness, there will be a somber white complexion.

This discussion covers the key symptoms and diagnostic methods of liver illnesses, although it does not cover them completely. There are still a great many symptoms that are commonly seen in liver illnesses such as headache, ocular redness, and tinnitus; however, they cannot all be discussed [in this essay].

3. ANALYSIS OF TREATMENT METHODS FOR LIVER ILLNESSES

The treatment methods employed in liver illnesses are rather complex. According to the *Nèi Jīng,* there are three principal therapeutic indicators pertaining to the liver:

1. The liver likes sour.

2. When the liver suffers, sweet foods relax it.

3. The liver likes to be dissipated, and acrid foods dissipate it, so use acrid to supplement it and sour to dissipate it.

We speak here of sour, sweet, and acrid as the flavors of medicinals selected to treat the liver. Sour and bitter are indicative of the nature of the liver viscus itself. By comparison, liver blood should be stored, moistened, and nourished; liver qi should be soothed and made patent. If internal-external factors that tend to stimulate pathological changes are encountered, then we should use medicinals for sour contracting, sweet relaxing, and acrid draining, because these treatment principles adjust the liver and help restore it to normal function. Therefore, in speaking of supplementation and draining here, we cannot simply generalize our explanation by saying, "if there is vacuity, supplement it, and if there is repletion, drain it."

---

[32]Fright wind, *jīng fēng:* disease occurring in infants and children, characterized by convulsive spasm and loss of consciousness. Fright wind is often loosely translated as infantile convulsions.

The implication is that if the medicinals are used appropriately to disinhibit the function of the liver viscus, then this therapy is supplementing; on the other hand, if medicinals are used inappropriately and inhibit the function of the liver viscus, then this has a draining effect. Although the principles of draining and supplementation are dissimilar, they have a single purpose, which is to supplement and return to normal. Therefore, sweet and sour are basically used to supplement the liver, but may be used to dissipate it; thus they can also have a harmful effect. This is why we say, "the liver likes sour," and, "sour drains it;" but we also say, "acrid dissipates it," and, "use acrid to supplement it."

In general, the essence of this idea begins in the physiology of the liver viscus itself and we must understand that regulation of the physiological function of the liver is of primary importance in the treatment of liver illnesses. In later times, the *Nàn Jīng* stated, "Where there is a detriment to the liver, moderate the middle." In the *Jīn Guì Yào Luè* it states:

> In liver illnesses, supplement with sour medicinals, assisted by burnt bitter medicinals. To augment this, use sweet-tasting medicinals to regulate it.

This quotation emphasizes that in fact the dose of bitter medicinals is also increased when treating liver illnesses. It is my belief that an integrated set of treatment principles is available to us based on the texts cited above.

The [following] treatment principles may be fixed as the four foundations for treatment of liver illnesses:

1. When supplementing the liver, use sour flavors.

2. When relaxing the liver, use sweet flavors.

3. When coursing the liver, use acrid flavors.

4. When clearing the liver, use bitter flavors. (The intention of the *Jīn Quì Yào Luè* differs in this regard.)

Based on this foundation, since the nature of any medicinal encompasses its qi, taste, ascending, or descending qualities and sinking or floating qualities, we may extend the therapeutic logic to produce different applications using [the above listed] medicinal compatibilities. These are sweet and sour to transform the yin; acrid and sweet to transform the yang; bitter and cold to drain fire; and sweet and cold to produce fluids. Furthermore, because of the relationships of engenderment and restraint within the five-phase relationships among the viscera, more indirect therapies are possible beyond the direct treatment of liver illnesses. These may include [methods such as] enriching the yin to nourish the liver and assisting metal to calm wood. Obviously, in clinical practice, the various applications of such treatment principles are rather complex, yet within their practices our predecessors continually summarized their experience, attempting to discover a set of useful clinical rules for the treatment of liver illnesses.

For example, Lǐ Guānxiān set forth the [following] ten principles:

1. Acrid is dissipating.

2. Sour is constraining.

3. Sweet is relaxing.

4. The heart is the son of the liver; if [the liver] is replete, then drain the son.

5. The kidney is the mother of the liver; if there is [a liver] vacuity, then supplement the mother.

6. The lung governs the qi; if liver qi counterflows, then clearing metal and downbearing the [qi of the] lung will calm it.

7. If there is a counterflow of qi, it may produce gallbladder fire; if the gallbladder fire is calmed, then the liver qi will be calmed accordingly.

8. For a hyperactive effulgence of liver yang, the yin should not be nourished; rather, shells are used to constrain it.

9. A liver illness is initially spleen repletion.

10. For repletion fire in the liver, if it is mild, use *Zuǒ Jīn Wǎn* (Left-Running Metal Pill); if it is severe, use *Lóng Dǎn Xiè Gān Tāng* (Gentian Liver-Draining Decoction).

These ten principles for the treatment of liver illnesses are neatly organized as cardinal principles.

Wǎng Xùegāo discussed liver treatments according to the three categories of liver qi, liver wind, and liver fire symptoms. Although many specific treatment principles have been advanced, in clinical practice he decided on those principles that were of guiding significance. In his approach the various aspects of liver qi are divided into the following categories: splenic insult, stomach exploitation, cardiac surge, pulmonary attack harboring cold, and vacuity of the root with repletion of the branch. He settled on [the following] eight treatment methods:

1. Methods for coursing the liver and regulating the qi are indicated when the liver qi, as the root channel, is depressed on its own, with qi distension producing bilateral costal pain. In such cases use medicinals such as *xiāng fù zǐ* (cyperus [root]), *yù jīn* (curcuma [tuber]), *zǐ sū gěng* (perilla stem), *qīng pí* (unripe tangerine peel) and *jú yè* (tangerine leaf). With simultaneous cold add *wú zhū yú* (evodia [fruit]), or with simultaneous heat add *mǔ dān pí* (moutan [root bark]) and *shān zhī zǐ* (gardenia [fruit]). Where there is simultaneous phlegm, add *bàn xià* (pinellia [tuber]) and *fú líng* (poria).

2. Methods for coursing the liver and freeing the network vessels are indicated when the qi will not respond to regulating [medicinals]. If there is obstruction of the constructive qi, or stasis blockage of the network vessels, then simultaneous freeing of the blood network vessels is indicated through the use of *xuán fù huā* (inula flower), *dāng guī* (tangkuei), *táo rén* (peach kernel) and *zé lán* (lycopus).

3. Methods for liver emolliation are used when there is an extreme distension of the liver qi, and excessive coursing of the liver also has [already] had an adverse effect.[33] The use of *dāng guī* (tangkuei), *gǒu*

---

[33]Trans: Excessive coursing of liver qi may be result from the nature of the disharmony or it may be iatrogenic.

qǐ zǐ (lycium [berry]), *bǎi zǐ rén* (biota seed) and *tǔ niú xī* (native achyranthes [root]) are indicated in these cases. With simultaneous heat, *mài mén dōng* (ophiopogon [tuber]) and *xiān dì huáng* (fresh rehmannia [root]) are added. With simultaneous cold, *ròu cōng róng* (cistanche [stem]) and *ròu guì* (cinnamon bark) are added.

4. Methods for relaxing the liver are indicated in the case of an exuberance of liver qi and vacuity of the middle burner. The use of *gān cǎo* (licorice [root]), *bái sháo yào* (white peony [root]), *suān zǎo rén* (spiny jujube [kernel]), *qīng pí* (unripe tangerine peel) and *mài yá* (barley sprout) is indicated.

5. Methods for banking up earth to drain wood are indicated in the case of liver qi overwhelming the spleen with gastric distension and pain. The use of *Liù Jūn Zǐ Tāng* (Six Gentlemen Decoction), with *wú zhū yú* (evodia [fruit]), *bái sháo yào* (white peony [root]) and *mù xiāng* (saussurea root), is indicated.

6. Methods for draining wood and harmonizing the stomach should be applied in the case of liver qi overwhelming the stomach with gastric pain and sour retching. The use of *Èr Chén Tang* (Two Matured Ingredients Decoction), *Zuǒ Jīn Wǎn* (Left-Running Metal Pill), *bái dòu kòu* (cardamom), and *chuān liàn zǐ* (toosendan [fruit]), is indicated.

7. Methods for draining the liver are indicated in the case of an upsurge of liver qi into the heart. Where there is heat reversal and cardiac pain, delete *huáng lián* (coptis [root]), and use *chuān liàn zǐ* (toosendan [fruit]) and *ròu guì* (cinnamon bark). If there are simultaneous chills and fever, include *huáng lián* (coptis [root]). [In such instances] *bái sháo yào* (white peony [root]) may also be added.[34]

8. Methods for repressing the liver are indicated in the case of an upsurge of liver qi into the lung, with sudden costal pain and violent ascension of qi and panting [dyspnea]. Use *sāng zhī* (mulberry twig) fried in the juice of *wú zhū yú* (evodia [fruit]), *zǐ sū gěng* (perilla stem), *xìng rén* (apricot kernel), and *jú hóng* (red tangerine peel).

In regard to liver wind, it is generally accepted that if [the symptoms are] at the vertex of the head, then the condition is mostly due to a hyperactivity of yang, and if [liver wind] affects the four limbs, it is primarily due to blood vacuity. Also, it is acknowledged that internal wind issues mainly from fire and that the common reference to a surplus of qi is actually fire. Five treatment principles have been settled on [by Wǎng]:

1. Methods for extinguishing wind and harmonizing the yang are those that cool the liver. When liver wind arises with the symptoms of mental and visual clouding and dizziness, use *líng yáng jiǎo* (antelope horn), *mǔ dān pí* (moutan [root bark]), *jú huā* (chrysanthemum [flower]), *gōu téng* (uncaria [stem and thorn]), *shí jué míng* (abalone shell) and *cì jí lí* (tribulus [fruit]).

---

[34]Trans: Keep in mind that Wǎng Xùegāo and Qin Bowei both assume that these treatment methods and medicinals are being applied within the context of a comprehensive treatment plan and a complete prescription.

2. Methods for extinguishing wind and subduing the yang are those that enrich the liver. If harmonizing the liver has been unsuccessful, use *mǔ lì* (oyster shell), *xiān dì huáng* (fresh rehmannia [root]), *nǚ zhēn zǐ* (ligustrum [fruit]), *xuán shēn* (scrophularia [root]), *bái sháo yào* (white peony [root]), *jú huā* (chrysanthemum [flower]) and *lù jiǎo jiāo* (deer-horn glue).

3. Methods for banking earth to settle wind are those that relax the liver. Where there is an upward counterflow of liver wind with a vacuity of the middle burner and little appetite, enrichment of the *yáng míng* is indicated along with drainage of the *jué yīn*. This is accomplished with the use of *rén shēn* (ginseng), *gān cǎo* (licorice [root]), *mài mén dōng* (ophiopogon [tuber]), *bái sháo yào* (white peony [root]), *jú huā* (chrysanthemum [flower]) and *yù zhú* (Solomon's seal [root]).

4. Methods for nourishing the liver address liver wind traveling in the extremities, with contracture and convulsion *[qiān zhì]* or numbness of the channels and network vessels. The use of *xiān dì huáng* (fresh rehmannia [root]), *dāng guī* (tangkuei), *gǒu qǐ zǐ* (lycium [berry]), *tǔ niú xī* (native achyranthes [root]), *tiān má* (gastrodia [root]), *hé shǒu wū* (flowery knotweed [root]), and *yǎ má rén* (flax seed) is indicated.

5. Methods for warming the liver are to be used in the case of severe vacuity wind cephalic dizziness and poor digestion. *Bái Zhú Fù Zǐ Tāng* (Ovate Atractylodes and Aconite Decoction) is indicated. Note that this supplements the middle [burner] rather than treating the liver directly.

In terms of liver fire, it is believed that as liver fire burns, it travels to the triple burner, the upper and lower, inner, and outer aspects of the entire body, all of which can become ill as a result of its spread through the triple burner. Ocular redness, malar flush, convulsions, mania, strangury stoppage, sores and ulcerations, hunger, thirst, nausea and vomiting, and insomnia are all symptoms of the overflow of blood above and below. Ten treatment methods have been settled on.

1. To clear the liver use *líng yáng jiǎo* (antelope horn), *mǔ dān pi* (moutan [root bark]), *shān zhī zǐ* (gardenia [fruit]), *huáng qín* (scutellaria [root]), *dàn zhú yè* (bamboo leaf), *lián qiáo* (forsythia [fruit]) and *xià kū cǎo* (prunella [spike]).

2. To drain the liver use prescriptions such as *Lóng Dǎn Xiè Gān Tāng* (Gentian Liver-Draining Decoction), *Xiè Qīng Wán* (Green-Blue-Draining Pill) and *Dāng Guī Lóng Huì Wán* (Tangkuei, Gentian, and Aloe Pill).

3. To clear metal to control wood in the case of an upward inflammation of liver fire that has been unsuccessfully cleared, use prescriptions such as *běi shā shēn* (glehnia [root]), *mài mén dōng* (ophiopogon [tuber]), *shí hú* (dendrobium [stem]), *pí pá yè* (loquat leaf), *tiān mén dōng* (asparagus [tuber]), *yù zhú* (Solomon's seal [root]) and *shí jué míng* (abalone shell).

4. To drain the son in the case of a repletion of liver fire, one must simultaneously drain the heart, thus *huáng lián* (coptis [root]) and *gān cǎo* (licorice [root]) are used.

5. To supplement the mother in the case of depletion of water and exuberance of fire, augment kidney water rather than use clearing techniques. [Augmenting kidney water is accomplished] with prescriptions such as *Liù Wèi Wán* (Six-Ingredient Pill) and *Dà Bǔ Yīn Wán* (Major Yin Supplementing Pill).

6. Transform the liver in cases with symptoms of depressive anger injuring the liver with a counterflow of qi mobilizing fire, vexation heat and costal pain, and distension fullness mobilizing the blood. The use of *qīng pí* (unripe tangerine peel), *mǔ dān pí* (moutan [root bark]), *shān zhī zǐ* (gardenia [fruit]), *bái sháo yào* (white peony [root]), *zé xiè* (alisma [tuber]), and *bèi mǔ* (fritillaria [bulb]) is indicated.

7. Warm the liver in the case of liver cold with an upward movement of qi characterized by sour vomiting. The use of *ròu guì* (cinnamon bark), *wú zhū yú* (evodia [fruit]), and *shǔ jiāo* (zanthoxylum husk) is indicated. With simultaneous central vacuity and a cold stomach, add *rén shen* (ginseng) and *gān jiāng* (dried ginger [root]).

8. To calm the liver use *chuān liàn zǐ* (toosendan [fruit]), *cì jí lí* (tribulus [fruit]), *gōu téng* (uncaria [stem and thorn]), and *jú yè* (tangerine leaf).

9. To dissipate the liver use *Xiāo Yáo Sǎn* (Free Wanderer Powder).

10. Track the liver where there is first internal wind, and later external wind develops. External wind may lead to a stirring of internal wind; thus liver wind is a miscellaneous category. Use *tiān má* (gastrodia [root]), *qiāng huó* (notopterygium [root]), *dú huó* (tuhuo [angelica root]), *bò hé* (mint), *màn jīng zǐ* (vitex [fruit]), *fáng fēng* (ledebouriella [root]), *bái jiāng cán* (silkworm), *chán tuì* (cicada molting), and *bái fù zǐ* (aconite/typhonium [tuber]).

Beyond this, the idea may still be advanced that regardless of whether the pattern is liver qi, liver wind, or liver fire, they all may be cured when the following seven treatment methods are used:

1. To supplement the liver use *hé shǒu wū* (flowery knotweed [root]), *tù sī zǐ* (cuscuta [seed]), *gǒu qǐ zǐ* (lycium [berry]), *suān zǎo rén* (spiny jujube [kernel]), *zhī má* (sesame [seed]), and *shā yuàn zǐ* (complanate astragalus seed).

2. To constrain the liver use *wū méi* (mume [fruit]), *bái sháo yào* (white peony [root]), and *mù guā* (chaenomeles [fruit]).

3. To calm the liver use *mǔ lì* (oyster shell), *shí jué míng* (abalone shell), *lóng gǔ* (dragon bone), *lóng chǐ* (dragon tooth), *dài zhě shí* (hematite), and *cí shí* (loadstone).

4. To supplement liver yin use *shú dì huáng* (cooked rehmannia [root]), *bái sháo yào* (white peony [root]), and *wū méi* (mume [fruit]).

5. To supplement liver yang use *ròu guì* (cinnamon bark), *shŭ jiāo* (zanthoxylum husk), and *ròu cōng róng* (cistanche [stem]).

6. To supplement liver blood use *dāng guī* (tangkuei), *xù duàn* (dipsacus [root]), *tŭ niú xī* (native achyranthes [root]), and *chuān xiōng* (ligusticum [root]).

7. To supplement liver qi use *tiān má* (gastrodia [root]), *bái sháo yào* (white peony [root]), *jú huā* (chrysanthemum [flower]), *shēng jiāng* (fresh ginger), *dù zhòng* (eucommia [bark]), *xì xīn* (asarum), and *yáng gān* (sheep liver).[35]

While the above treatment methods relate to Wăng Xùegāo's treatment of liver qi, liver wind, and liver fire, in fact they encompass the entire scope of treatment for liver illnesses. Through experiential analysis[36] we may conclude that these methods are of practical value in the clinic and must be given serious attention. To promote a good grasp of their use as clinical guides, I would like to propose some guiding principles of my own to promote further study.

First, the vacuity or repletion, cold or heat of the liver illness itself must be considered, that is, patterns such as insufficiency of liver blood, liver qi, or liver fire, surging counterflow, or hepatic contraction of pathogenic cold, and so forth. These are the most common liver illnesses, [therefore they] also [represent] the etiological and pathological dynamics of primary importance. Thus the treatment of these most common illnesses provides the foundation for the treatment of all liver illnesses.

Next, we must consider that more than one pathological change may simultaneously develop within a single pattern. For instance, a vacuity of liver blood and a scorching of liver heat may stir liver yang and a horizontal counterflow may enable an attack of the stomach and constrain the spleen. Although in these examples it is the liver yang and stomach-spleen symptoms that represent the primary etiology, it is nonetheless already apparent that in treatment simultaneous consideration should be given to both heat and vacuity.

Next, the relationship of the liver viscus with the other internal viscera must be considered, such as the capacity for water to engender wood and the fact that relaxing the middle may supplement the liver, and so forth. This, aside from being an indirect treatment of the liver, enables us to obtain an even greater agility in treatment.

In summary we can say that in considering these three aspects, it will not be difficult to differentiate the complexities of liver illnesses into primary and secondary concerns, nor is it difficult to use the branch and root principle to determine the priority, urgency, and sequence of therapies.

It was Wăng Xùegāo, for example, who advanced this treatment principle in his statement that supplementing liver blood, supplementing liver qi, supplementing liver yang, and supplementing liver yin are all principles for the treatment of liver vacuity; that calming the liver, dissipating the liver, coursing the liver and rectifying qi, and coursing the liver and

---

[35]Trans: *yáng gān* is also used for goat liver.

[36]Trans: The words Qin uses here, "experimental analysis," refer to his personal clinical experience, not clinical trials or biomedical assays as these words might imply in English.

freeing the network vessels are all principles for treating liver repletion; also, warming the liver is a principle for the treatment of liver cold, and clearing the liver and draining the liver are principles for the treatment of liver heat. Furthermore, draining the liver, constraining the liver, banking earth to drain wood, and banking earth to settle wind are all treatment principles that may be used concurrently. Finally, draining the son, supplementing the mother to warm earth, and clearing metal to control wood are all treatment principles pertaining to the use of the five-phase cycles of generation and restraint.

Although I recognize that these treatment methods are all based on distinct symptom patterns, there are still many individual terms that actually mean the same thing. Furthermore, some of the terms [that are commonly] used are not sufficiently defined, however these terms nonetheless maintain an intimate relationship with the use of medicinals in composition. Thus, a fresh arrangement [of these methods] is essential [to clinical clarity].

Supplementation of the Liver, Nourishment of the Liver, and Enrichment of the Liver

The liver stores the blood. In the case of vacuity, methods of enrichment, moistening, supplementation, and nourishment are indicated. Therefore we use the terms supplementation, nourishment, and enrichment. However, the clinical objective of these three methods is the same, and they are all treatment methods applied for an insufficiency of liver blood.

Emolliating the Liver, Relaxing the Liver, and Harmonizing the Liver

The liver is a dominating viscus and its nature is bitter and harsh. In pathological conditions this typically manifests as an upward counterflow of liver qi and an upward surging of liver fire. Emolliation is appropriate to constrain the domination; sweetness is appropriate to relax the harshness and to harmonize and disinhibit. Therefore, we call this emolliation, relaxation, and harmonization. Nonetheless, these treatment methods are mostly used for liver qi patterns where an exuberance of liver fire is absent, and where the liver qi pattern is from an essential blood vacuity. Therefore, the implication here is that of regulation and nourishment.

Constraining the Liver

In blood vacuity the blood is not subdued and stored. Thus it transforms into an upward harassment of wind. The middle should be enriched and nourished, assisted by sour astriction. This [method] will cause an abundance of yin that enables a spontaneous astriction of yang, [and] the wind will also be spontaneously extinguished. In general, if the symptoms of liver yang and liver wind are serious, we use supplementing medicines with a bias toward those medicines that also have enriching, slimy, and rich tastes.

Settling the Liver [Zhèn Gān]

This treatment method is also used for liver yang and liver wind. The objective is to subdue the yang and extinguish the wind, and, because the [implication of this] treatment is settling and quieting, it is referred to as "settling." In general, this method is often used with liver heat leading to stirring of liver wind, yet it differs from repressing the liver.[37]

Tracking the Liver

This method is used in treating liver illnesses characterized by mixed external and internal wind traveling to the orifices, channels, and network vessels. It is useful for tracking and eliminating pathogens, so it is referred to as "tracking." It is of primary importance in treating the penetration and protracted lingering of external wind. If the condition is purely one of internal wind, then this method is inappropriate.

Soothing the Liver, Dispersing the Liver, and Transforming the Liver

This treatment method is used for any depressive binding, blockage, or stagnation of liver qi and blood. In the case of depression, soothing is indicated. In the case of binding, dissipation is indicated, and in the case of blockage and stagnation, transformation is indicated to promote restoration of the liver's normal nature of orderly reaching. We therefore speak of "soothing," "dissipating," and "transforming." This is typically used in simultaneous vacuity and repletion patterns where the qi and blood are simultaneously affected, particularly where there are vacuity symptoms in the blood aspect.

Calming the Liver, Discharging the Liver, and Coursing the Liver

This treatment method is used for patterns of horizontal counterflow of liver qi, with distension and fullness and pi oppression. It is applied in order to calm, discharge, and course and drain, and therefore we speak of "calming," " discharging," and "coursing."

Repressing the Liver

This treatment method is also used for the treatment of liver qi patterns. Because its attendant manifestation is surging counterflow, which must additionally be repressed and controlled, it is termed repression.

Clearing the Liver and Cooling the Liver

This treatment method is applied in the case of both an internal depression of liver heat and an internal harassment of liver fire. It is equally appropriate to use cooling prescriptions to clear [the heat or fire]. Therefore we speak of "clearing" and "cooling."

Draining the Liver [*Xiè Gān*]

In the case of an upward harassment of liver fire, the foundation [treatment] for clearing the liver must go one step further by using bitter cold medicines for directly breaking and draining the fire. Therefore, we say this is "draining."

---

[37]Trans: While methods for repressing the liver and settling the liver are both oriented toward addressing an ascension of yang and wind, they differ in their approach to the problem. Methods for repressing the liver imply supplementing blood/yin, which in addressing the root of the yang wind will spontaneously arrest it. Methods for settling the liver imply direct subducting of the yang wind. In the case of repression, medicinals such as *guī bǎn* (tortoise plastron) are used, while in the case of settling the liver, medicinals such as *gōu téng* (uncaria [stem and thorn]) and *shí jué míng* (abalone shell) are used. Repressing methods are fundamentally nutritive while settling methods are fundamentally sedative in nature.

Warming the Liver

When pathogenic cold injures the liver, it is appropriate to use warming prescriptions that are acrid and dissipating. When there is an insufficiency of yang qi within the liver viscus itself, it is appropriate to warm, nourish, and help promote qi and its development. [In both cases the method] is generally called "warming"; however it has two different meanings.

In general, the names for these treatment methods have been decided based on pathological changes within the liver viscus itself. The specific presentation of the pathological changes such as liver qi, liver fire, liver yang, and liver wind, and so forth, also must be stressed in treatment. As a result of this emphasis we have additional names for treatment methods. For instance [there are the the following]:

Coursing the Qi, Rectifying the Qi, Regulating the Qi, and Soothing the Qi

It is appropriate to course and smooth liver qi, regardless of whether there is horizontal counterflow or depressive binding. Liver function should be regulated by soothing and disinhibing. Thus we speak of coursing, regulating, and soothing. As for calming the liver, discharging the liver, and coursing the liver, these terms all mean the same thing.

Clearing Heat and Clearing Fire

If it is mild, it is heat. If it is severe and flares upward, it is fire. This encompasses vacuity heat and vacuity fire as well; thus cold, cooling, and clearing [treatment methods] are indicated, so we speak of "clearing." The therapeutic implications of cooling and clearing the liver are the same.

Descending Fire and Draining Fire

In the case of an unchecked flaring of liver fire, direct and forceful downbearing or downward draining is indicated, so we speak of downbearing and draining, each of which pertains to the class of [methods that treat] repletion. Draining the liver means the same thing.

Subduing the Yang

An upward harassment of liver yang is mainly due to blood vacuity and the subsequent rising of blood heat. Treatment by subduing and storing is indicated; therefore we speak of "subduing." Calming the liver means the same thing.

Extinguishing Wind

When liver wind is severe as contrasted to the pattern of liver yang, treatment by calming and extinguishing, calming, and clearing is indicated. Therefore, we speak of "extinguishing." Calming the liver and constraining the liver [liǎn gān] mean the same thing.

Tracking Wind

When internal wind and external wind suddenly enter the orifices, the channels, and the network vessels, it must be sought and dissipated. Therefore we speak of "tracking." Tracking the liver means the same thing.

The meanings of these treatment methods are the same as those discussed in the fundamental work presented above. The most important fact is that they develop from the liver viscus itself. The clinical presentation of the pathological changes is primary in the discrimination of the above parameters. Nonetheless, when writing a prescription, these methods are most commonly combined. For instance, methods for calming the liver are combined with methods for regulating the qi; methods for clearing the liver are combined with those for descending fire; methods for calming are combined with those for constraining the yang; methods for subduing the liver are combined with methods for extinguishing wind, and so forth. I believe that if treatment methods are combined in this manner, we eliminate duplication among the functions of the herbs in a prescription and they will more accurately reflect the pathological mechanisms. Nonetheless the meanings [of each term] must be thoroughly understood.

Chart One

The Relationships of Pathologies and Treatment Methods

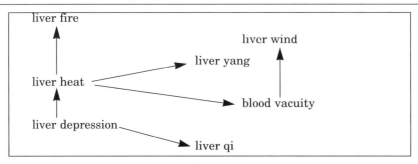

Chart Two: Liver Pathologies

Liver Blood

Treatment Methods	Medicinals	Formula
Supplementation, nourishment, and enrichment of the liver	*bái sháo yào* (white peony [root]) *shú dì huáng* (cooked rehmannia [root])	*Sì Wù Tāng* (Four Agents Decoction)

Blood vacuity causing upward harassment of wind

Treatment Methods	Medicinals	Formula
Repressing the liver	*guī bǎn* (tortoise plastron)	*Zhèn Gān Xī Fēng Tāng* (Liver-Settling Wind-Extinguishing Decoction)

Liver yang; Liver wind

Treatment Methods	Medicinals	Formula
Settling the liver	*gōu tén* (uncaria [stem and thorn])	*Tiān Má Gān Téng Yǐn* (Gastrodia and Uncaria Beverage)

Mixed internal external wind

Treatment Methods	Medicinals	Formula
Tracking liver wind	*wú gōng* (centipede)	*Zhǐ Jìng Gōng Sǎn* (Tetany-Resolving Powder)

Depressive binding; Stasis of liver qi and blood

Treatment Methods	Medicinals	Formula
Soothing, dispersing, and transforming the liver	*xiāng fù zǐ* (cyperus [root]	*Xiāo Yáo Sǎn* (Free Wanderer Powder)

Depression of heart and liver fire

Treatment Methods	Medicinals	Formula
Clearing the liver Cooling the liver	*lóng dǎn* (gentian [root]), *xià kū cǎo* (prunella [spike]), *huáng qín* (scutellaria [root])	*Lóng Dǎn Xiè Gān Tāng* (Gentian Liver-Draining Decoction)

Liver fire

Treatment Methods	Medicinals	Formula
Draining liver fire	*dǎn cǎo* (gentian [root])	*Zhì Qīng Wán* (Green-Blue Draining Pill)

Pathogenic cold; Insufficiency of yang

Treatment Methods	Medicinals	Formula
Warming the liver	*wú zhū* (evodia[fruit]), *ròu guì* (cinnamon bark), *yín yáng huò* (epimedium)	*Jiāo Ài Tāng* Ass Hide Glue and Mugwort Decoction

4. ON THE USE OF COMMONLY USED PRESCRIPTIONS FOR LIVER ILLNESSES

The cardinal principles exemplified in the commonly used prescriptions for liver illnesses are those of nourishing the blood, harmonizing the blood, regulating the qi, and downbearing the fire. Because of the complexity of the possible changes in etiology and pathomechanism, modifications are made according to the symptoms, and very few prescriptions are fixed. The primary etiologies and symptoms are apparent in the established prescriptions that treat liver illnesses. When researching prescriptions for liver illnesses, it is essential to incorporate the experience of our predecessors in using medicinals in prescription. Thus they may be used with agility in the clinic and these standard prescriptions will be effectively utilized rather than fettering [our treatment strategies]. We will now select some commonly used prescriptions with which to explain these issues.

Sì Wù Tāng (Four Agents Decoction)	
from *Hé Jì Jú Fāng*	
shú dì huáng	cooked rehmannia [root]
bái sháo yào	white peony [root]
dāng guī	tangkuei
chuān xiōng	ligusticum [root]

This is a prescription of general use[38] for supplementing and harmonizing the blood. Its application is not limited to liver illnesses. Because the liver governs blood storage, this formula has a relatively large number of uses in the treatment of blood vacuity and it is the primary prescription for supplementing the liver.

The combination of *shú dì huáng* (cooked rehmannia [root]) and *bái sháo yào* (white peony [root]) in this prescription are the blood within the blood medicinals, where *dāng guī* (tangkuei) and *chuān xiōng* (ligusticum [root]) are the qi within the blood medicinals. The activity of yin and yang is combined and this therefore enables supplementation and harmonization of the blood. If only *dì huáng* and *chuān xiōng* are used, this protects without moving. If only *dāng guī* and *chuān xiōng* are used, this moves without protecting. This variation with *dāng guī* is known as *Xiōng Guī Sǎn* (Ligusticum and Tangkuei Powder), but is also called *Fó Shǒu Sǎn* (Hand-of-Buddha Powder). It frees the menses and eliminates stasis. It is an obvious example of the therapeutic variations of an established prescription.

In general, when nourishing the blood and harmonizing the blood in liver illnesses, the enriching and slimy *shú dì huáng* (cooked rehmannia [root]) is often left out. There is a bias among clinicians toward the use of acrid medicinals such as *chuān xiōng* (ligusticum [root]) and particularly *dāng guī* (tangkuei) and *bái sháo yào* (white peony [root]). Our predecessors used modifications of *Sì Wù Tāng* (Four Agents Decoction) as the foremost prescription for treating liver illnesses. For instance, in *Yī Zōng Jīn Jiàn Fāng*, an insufficiency of liver yin and dizziness causing collapse is treated by *Bǔ Gān Sǎn* (Liver-Supplementing Powder), which is comprised of *mài mén dōng* (ophiopogon [tuber]), *suān zǎo rén* (spiny jujube [kernel]), *mù guā* (chaenomeles [fruit]), and *gān cao* (licorice [root]), all of which are added to the source prescription, *Sì Wù Tāng* (Four Agents Decoction).

An abundance of liver-gallbladder fire coercing wind heat was also treated by *Chái Hú Qīng Gān Yǐn* (Bupleurum Liver-Clearing Beverage), which is comprised of *huáng qín* (scutellaria [root]), *lián qiáo* (forsythia [fruit]), *shān zhī zǐ* (gardenia [fruit]), *niú bàng zǐ* (arctium [seed]), *fáng fēng* (ledebouriella [root]), *tiān huā fěn* (trichosanthes root), and *gān cǎo* (licorice [root]), added to the source prescription.

Zī Shuǐ Qīng Gān Yǐn (Water-Enriching Liver-Clearing Beverage)	
from *Yī Zōng Jǐ Rèn Piān*	
shú dì huáng	cooked rehmannia [root]
shān zhū yú	cornus [fruit]
shān yào	dioscorea [root]
mǔ dān pí	moutan [root bark]
fú líng	poria
zé xiè	alisma [tuber]
chái hú	bupleurum [root]
bái sháo yào	white peony [root]
shān zhī zǐ	gardenia [fruit]
suān zǎo rén	spiny jujube [kernel]

[40]Here, "general use" is a technical term relating to the primary patterns addressed by a formula. See "On the skillful utilization of established prescriptions" in the following section.

The base prescription is related to *Liù Wèi Dì Huáng Tāng* (Six-Ingredient Rehmannia Decoction) with additions, and is indicated for insufficiency of kidney yin and vacuity dryness of liver blood, simultaneously accompanied by symptoms of internal depression of fire qi such as remittent fever, intercostal qi stasis, and vomiting of sour fluid. Therefore, *bái sháo yào* (white peony [root]), *chái hú* (bupleurum [root]), and *shān zhī zǐ* (gardenia [fruit]), are added to the foundation of enriching the kidney to nourish the liver, protect liver yin, course liver qi, and clear liver fire. In the case of liver vacuity, there will be gallbladder timidity influencing sleep and frequent palpitations. *Suān zǎo rén* (spiny jujube [kernel]) is therefore added to calm the spirit.

Liù Wèi Dì Huáng Tāng (Six-Ingredient Rehmannia Decoction) is the base prescription for enriching the kidney. The liver is the son of the kidney; where there is liver vacuity, supplement the mother. Therefore, this forumla is typically used with liver vacuity symptoms.

Líng Yáng Jiǎo Tāng (Antelope Horn Decoction)	
from *Tōng Sǔ Shāng Hán Lùn*	
líng yáng jiǎo	antelope horn
gōu téng	uncaria [stem and thorn]
dì huáng	raw rehmannia [root]
bái sháo yào	white peony [root]
sāng yè	mulberry leaf
bèi mǔ	fritillaria [bulb]
jú huā	chrysanthemum [flower]
fú líng	poria
gān cǎo	licorice [root]
zhú rú	bamboo shavings

This prescription was originally used to treat pathogenic heat entering the *jué yīn,* with a consequent clouding of the spirit and convulsions *[chōu chù].* Since extreme heat injures the yin, wind is stirred and phlegm generated. The spirit is not calm and there is a hypertonicity of the sinew vessels. Therefore, *líng yáng jiǎo* (antelope horn), *gōu téng* (uncaria [stem and thorn]), *sāng yè* (mulberry leaf), and *jú huā* (chrysanthemum [flower]) are the main ingredients used to cool the liver and extinguish wind. They are assisted by *xiān dì huáng* (fresh rehmannia [root]), *bái sháo yào* (white peony [root]), and *gān cǎo* (licorice [root]), which are sweet and sour and transform the yin, enrich the fluids and relax urgency. *Bèi mǔ* fritillaria [bulb], *zhú rú* (bamboo shavings), and *fú líng* (poria) transform phlegm and free the network vessels, clear the heart, and calm the spirit. Because there is an ascending counterflow of liver heat, wind, or yang in this liver illness, and the pathomechanisms are identical, this prescription is also typically used with severe symptoms of liver yang, counterflow of liver heat and wind yang; *shí jué míng* (abalone shell) [and so forth] also may be included to constrain and calm liver yang.[39]

---

[39]Trans: Other medicinals such as *mǔ lì* (oyster shell) and *lóng gǔ* (dragon bone) may also be included.

Dà Dìng Fēng Zhū (Major Wind-Stabilizing Pill)	
from *Wēn Bìng Tiáo Biàn*	
bái sháo yào	white peony [root]
ē jiāo	ass hide glue
guī bǎn	tortoise plastron
xiān dì huáng	fresh rehmannia [root]
huǒ má rén	hemp seed
wǔ wèi zǐ	schisandra [berry]
mǔ lì	oyster shell
biē jiǎ	turtle shell
mài mén dōng	ophiopogon [tuber]
gān cǎo	baked licorice [root]
jī nèi jīn	gizzard lining
jī dǎn	chicken's gallbladder

This prescription treats pathogenic warm heat dissipating the true yin, presenting as lassitude and excitability, a weak pulse with a crimson tongue, and occasionally vacuity desertion. Therefore, a large group of medicinals for enriching the yin are used, assisted by shells to constrain the yang as well as to calm and settle it. In liver illnesses where extreme vacuity of liver and kidney yin and blood are encountered, there is an incessant agitation of internal wind with symptoms of dizziness and myopia, tinnitus, twitching and spasms of the sinew and muscle, and an unsettled mind that brims over with thoughts. In these cases, this prescription is modified.

Whenever there is an ascending harassment of wind yang with a great vacuity of liver yin, presenting as water not containing wood, *bái sháo yào* (white peony [root]) and *xiān dì huáng* (fresh rehmannia [root]) are typically used to treat the root, and are combined with other medicinals to extinguish wind and settle the yang. Nonetheless, it is appropriate to cool and calm the liver yang, and liver wind must be supplemented [in order to be extinguished]. The depth of understanding in the use of these medicinals may be seen by contrasting this prescription with *Líng Yáng Jiǎo Tāng* (Antelope Horn Decoction).[40]

Zhēn Zhū Mǔ Wán (Mother-of-Pearl Pill)	
from *Běn Shù Fāng*	
zhēn zhū	pearl Margarita
shú dì huáng	cooked rehmannia [root]
rén shēn	ginseng
dāng guī	tangkuei
xī jiǎo	rhinoceros horn
chén xiāng	aquilaria [wood]
lóng chǐ	dragon tooth
suān zǎo rén	spiny jujube [kernel]
bǎi zǐ rén	biota seed
fú líng	poria
administered in honey pills covered with *zhū shā* (cinnabar)	

---

[40]There are some subtle differences between *Dà Dìng Fēng Zhū* (Major Wind-Stabilizing Pill) and *Líng Yáng Jiǎo Tāng* (Antelope Horn Decoction). Both address an attack of pathogenic heat; however, the use of *líng yáng jiǎo* (antelope horn) and *gōu téng* (uncaria [stem and thorn]) as the sovereign medicinals in *Líng Yáng Jiǎo Tāng* place its emphasis primarily on settling the yang. The other ingredients in this prescription address yin vacuity and phlegm. *Dà Dìng Fēng Zhū*, on the other hand, with its heavy use of cloying medicinals that enrich the yin, primarily addresses the injury to the true yin incurred from the pathogenic heat.

The root prescription treats insufficiency of liver blood and internal stirring of wind yang, with symptoms of dizziness, flowery vision, restless sleep, palpitations, and a weak and fine pulse. The *rén shēn* (ginseng), *dāng guī* (tangkuei), and *shú dì huáng* (cooked rehmannia [root]) are employed to bank up and nourish the root source of the liver and kidney. *Zhēn zhū* (pearl Margarita) is heavy and contrains the yang, and is assisted by medicinals identified as calming the spirit. It should be noted that the aspects of calming and constraining the yang are clearly emphasized by including *zhēn zhū* (pearl Margarita) in the title of the prescription. The source text comments, "True Margarita is larger than [common] Margarita and is irregularly shaped." It also states, "Take three fen of unpowdered *zhēn zhū*, grind it to the consistency of flour, and administer." It is understood that "true Margarita" is powdered *zhēn zhū* which simultaneously enriches the yin, but which is different from the *zhēn zhū* commonly used today.

Sāng Má Wán (Mulberry Leaf and Sesame Pill)

from *Hú Zēng Fāng*

sāng yè	mulberry leaf
zhī má	sesame [seed]

[These medicinals are] made into honey pills.

Sesame nourishes the blood, while mulberry leaf clears heat. The prescription is thus extremely simple. Nonetheless, it supplements the liver and boosts the kidney, cools the blood, and eliminates wind. It is generally used for liver yang headache and dizziness. It has the function of enriching below while clearing above and is quite effective. If the stools tend toward dryness, then simultaneously use it with *Rùn Cháng Tāng* (Intestine-Moistening Decoction).

Xiǎo Chái Hú Tāng (Minor Bupleurum Decoction)

from *Shāng Hán Lùn*

chái hú	bupleurum [root]
huáng qín	scutellaria [root]
rén shēn	ginseng
bàn xià	pinellia [tuber]
shēng jiāng	fresh ginger
zhì gān cǎo	mix-fried licorice [root]
dà zǎo	jujube

The base prescription treats pathogenic injury by cold that transforms and enters the *shào yáng* with symptoms such as intermittent chills and fever, thoracocostal fullness, vexation and nausea, and a wiry pulse. This prescription is not [strictly speaking] a prescription for liver illnesses. Because intermittent fever and chills may appear within the context of a liver illness, it is typically used in those cases; however, we must understand that this implies modification of the root prescription.

The essential aim in the organization of *Xiǎo Chái Hú Tāng* (Minor Bupleurum Decoction) is to support the correct and reach the pathogen. Because the external pathogen has transformed and entered the *shào yáng*, resolution of the exterior is indicated. *Chái hú* (bupleurum [root]) evicts the pathogen in the *shào yáng* and *huáng qín* (scutellaria [root]) clears the heat of *shào yáng*. Also, because internal symptoms appear, these [medicinals] are assisted by *bàn xià* (pinellia [tuber]) and *shēng jiāng* (fresh ginger) to harmonize the stomach and *rén shēn* (ginseng), *gān cǎo* (licorice [root]), and *dà zǎo* (jujube) to bank up the middle. This makes it clear that the illness is in the qi aspect and not in the blood aspect.

In terms of modifications, if there is vexation heat in the chest without vomiting, with heat gradually transforming to dryness, delete the *bàn xià* (pinellia [tuber]) and *rén shēn* (ginseng) and add *guā lóu* (trichosanthes [fruit]) to actually generate fluids. If there is abdominal pain with an insult to stomach yang, delete the *huáng qín* (scutellaria [root]) and add *bái sháo yào* (white peony [root]) to constrain wood. For subcostal lump glomus and horizontal counterflow of liver qi, delete the *dà zǎo* (jujube) and add *mǔ lì* (oyster shell), which is salty and softening.

The above symptoms clarify the indications for the use of *Xiāo Chái Hú Tāng* (Minor Bupleurum Decoction). In liver illness, one must discriminate whether [the pathology] is in the qi or the blood, whether there is or is not heat, and whether the stomach and spleen are vacuous or replete. If, on the other hand, it is in the blood, there is no heat, and the spleen and stomach are replete, [then] the *Xiǎo Chái Hú Tāng* is contraindicated.[41]

Sì Nì Sǎn (Counterflow Cold Powder)	
from *Shāng Hán Lùn*	
chái hú	bupleurum [root]
bái sháo yào	white peony [root]
zhǐ ké	bitter orange
gān cǎo	baked licorice [root]

This prescription treats the transmission of pathogenic heat with symptoms of reversal counterflow of the limbs from an internal depression of yang qi, which is therefore called "four counterflows." Because *chái hú* (bupleurum [root]) and *zhǐ ké* (bitter orange) are used together, they are able to upbear the clear and downbear the turbid. The *bái sháo yào* (white peony [root]) and *zhǐ ké* (bitter orange) are used together to smoothe qi stasis. Together the *bái sháo yào* (white peony [root]) and *gān cǎo* (licorice [root]) relax urgency and relieve pain. In general the prescription functions to course the liver and rectify the spleen, regulate the qi and eliminate stasis, and therefore it is commonly used in the treatment of liver illnesses. Later on, *Chái Hú Shū Gān Sǎn* (Bupleurum Liver-Coursing Powder) evolved from this prescription.

I believe that in the treatment of liver illnesses in general the use of *Xiǎo Chái Hú Tāng* (Minor Bupleurum Decoction) is inferior to the use of *Sì Nì Sǎn* (Counterflow Cold Powder), which is not only oriented toward coursing the liver but which is also free from [the potential] side effects [of *Xiāo Chái Hú Tāng* (Minor Bupleurum Decoction)]. The addition of *dāng guī* (tangkuei) and *qīng pí* (unripe tangerine peel) may be incorporated into the prescription to treat liver depression causing disharmonious stomach qi. *Qīng pí* may be added for costal pain.

---

[41]Trans: In other words, this prescription is appropriate when the illness is in the qi aspect, where there is heat and spleen-stomach vacuity.

Although this is similar to *Xiāo Yáo Sǎn* (Free Wanderer Powder), in reality they have distinct [therapeutic applications]. This is because *Xiāo Yáo Sǎn* uses *cāng zhú* (atractylodes [root]), *fú líng* (poria), and *gān cǎo* (licorice [root]) in addition to *dāng guī* (tangkuei), *bái sháo yào* (white peony [root]), and *chái hú* (bupleurum [root]) with the intent to supplement the liver and strengthen the spleen. Here [in Counterflow Cold Powder], *cāng zhú* (atractylodes [root]) and *fú líng* (poria) are deleted and replaced by *zhǐ ké* (bitter orange) and *qīng pí* (unripe tangerine peel), placing the focus on harmonizing the stomach. Thus the intent of each prescription is quite different.

Chái Hú Shū Gān Sǎn (Bupleurum Liver-Coursing Powder)	
from *Jǐng Yuè Quán Shū*	
chái hú	bupleurum [root]
bái sháo yào	white peony [root]
chuān xiōng	ligusticum [root]
zhǐ ké	bitter orange
xiāng fù zǐ	cyperus [root]
gān cǎo	baked licorice [root]
chén pí	tangerine peel

This prescription is comprised of *Sì Nì Sǎn* (Counterflow Cold Powder) with the additions of *chuān xiōng* (ligusticum [root]), *xiāng fù zǐ* (cyperus [root]), and *chén pí* (tangerine peel) to harmonize the blood and regulate the qi in the treatment of costal pain and intermittent fever and chills with the aim of coursing the liver. Coursing the liver is primarily aimed at regulating the qi, but it is not appropriate to circulate the qi excessively. Furthermore, we must consider the liver itself and we cannot simply regulate the qi and ignore the other factors that might be involved. In this prescription, *chái hú* (bupleurum [root]), *zhǐ ké* (bitter orange), *xiāng fù zǐ* (cyperus [root]), and *chén pí* (tangerine peel) are the main ingredients for regulating the qi. These are assisted by *bái sháo yào* (white peony [root]) and *chuān xiōng* (ligusticum [root]), which harmonize the blood. *Gān cǎo* (baked licorice [root]) is used as a mediator. This is the central method of coursing the liver and it has come to be considered a skillful adaption of an ancient prescription.[42]

Jiě Gān Qiān (Liver-Resolving Brew)	
from *Jǐng Yuè Quán Shū*	
bái sháo yào	white peony [root]
zǐ sū yè	perilla leaf
bàn xià	pinellia [tuber]
chén pí	tangerine peel
bái dòu kòu	cardamom
hòu pò	magnolia bark
fú líng	poria

This prescription is called "resolving the liver." In fact, with the exception of *bái sháo yào* (white peony [root]), which supplements the liver, and

---

[42]Trans: It should be noted that the prepared formula named *Shū Gān Wán* (Liver-Soothing Pills) is a different formulation than *Chái Hú Shū Gān Sǎn* (Bupleurum Liver-Coursing Powder).

zǐ sū yè (perilla leaf), which is at the same time a fragrant qi soother, all the medicinals belong to the categories of dampness transforming, stasis moving and stomach and spleen regulating medicinals. These are all medicinals that address symptoms of blockage of earth and depression of wood. Because qi stasis causing damp obstruction of the stomach and spleen influences the orderly extension of liver qi, the root treatment must emphasize the middle burner. Therefore, the prescription does not contain *chái hú* (bupleurum [root]) but rather utilizes *zǐ sū yè* (perilla leaf), which is chosen for its capacity to soothe liver depression as well as its capacity to harmonize the stomach and spleen. With the spleen and stomach healthy and motile, liver qi becomes uninhibited on its own. Therefore, the implication of [the name] "liver-resolving" is actually that of resolving the areas surrounding and influenced by the liver, and not that of directly treating the liver itself. Clinically, when a liver illness produces slow digestion, abdominal distension, and spleen stomach symptoms, which are relatively severe, this prescription should be used first to harmonize the middle.

Huà Gān Jiān (Liver-Transforming Brew)
from *Jǐng Yuè Quán Shū*

bái sháo yào	white peony [root]
qīng pí	unripe tangerine peel
chén pí	tangerine peel
mǔ dān pí	moutan [root bark]
shān zhī zǐ	gardenia [fruit]
bèi mǔ	fritillaria [bulb]
zé xiè	alisma [tuber]

This prescription focuses heavily on the [direct] treatment of the liver, employing *bái sháo yào* (white peony [root]) to protect liver yin, and *qīng pí* (unripe tangerine peel) to course liver qi, as well as *mǔ dān pí* (moutan [root bark]) and *shān zhī zǐ* (gardenia [fruit]) to clear liver fire. It is indicated for thoracocostal fullness and pain due to an internal depression of fire qi in the liver viscus. It is also indicated for symptoms of coughing of phlegm and blood, all from an upward counterflow of qi fire attacking the lung. Because qi fire may cause a blockage of phlegm dampness, *bèi mǔ* (fritillaria [bulb]) and *zé xiè* (alisma [tuber]) are therefore added. *Bèi mǔ* is used for its simultaneous effect of resolving depression of qi.

Yuè Jú Wán (Depression-Overcoming Pill)
from *Dān Xī Xīn Fǎ*

cāng zhú	atractylodes [root]
xiāng fù zǐ	cyperus [root]
chuān xiōng	ligusticum [root]
shān zhī zǐ	gardenia [fruit]
shén qū	medicated leaven

The main thrust of this prescription is moving the qi and resolving its depression in a general way, and as such it is not primarily a liver qi pescription. The prescription uses *cāng zhú* (atractylodes [root]) to resolve depressive dampness, *xiāng fù zǐ* (cyperus [root]) to resolve depressive qi, *chuān xiōng* (ligusticum [root]) to resolve depression of the blood, *shān zhī zǐ* (gardenia [fruit]) to resolve depressive fire, and *shén qū* (medicated leaven) to resolve digestate depression. Since the qi is circulated and the dampness removed, the untransformed phlegm is spontaneously resolved. Therefore, illnesses of all six depressions may be treated with only five medicinals.

The primary etiology of the six depressions begins with qi stasis, then damp digestate, phlegm fire, and blood become mutually encumbered, and then depressed. Nonetheless, it is not a case of one depression engendering six, rather they are all [six simultaneously] depressed. Furthermore, each of the six depressions may be either mild or severe relative to one another and they should not be treated in the same way. Therefore, medicinals should be divided into primary and secondary classes and the root prescription modified. For instance, if depressive qi is particularly severe, then add *mù xiāng* (saussurea [root]). If depressive dampness tends to be severe, then add *fú líng* (poria). If depressive blood is severe, then add *hóng huā* (carthamus [flower]). If depressive fire is severe, then add *dà qīng yè* (isatis leaf). If digestate depression is severe, then add *bái dòu kòu* (cardamom). For copious phlegm, add *bàn xià* (pinellia [tuber]); and for harassment of cold add *wú zhū yú* (evodia [fruit]), and so forth.

Whenever we research and use standard prescriptions, we must try to understand the theory and practice of our predecessors. For instance, Zhū Dānxī explicitly noted that all qi depression pertains to the lung. He also recognized that most depressive qi illnesses were located in the middle burner, involving the loss of the respective capacities for upbearing and downbearing within the spleen and stomach. If we mistake the resolution of depressive qi in general for soothing the liver qi in particular, this misses Zhū Dānxī's original intent.

Xiāo Yáo Sǎn (Free Wanderer Powder)	
from *Hé Jì Jú Fāng*	
chái hú	bupleurum [root]
dāng guī	tangkuei
bái sháo yào	white peony [root]
cāng zhú	atractylodes [root]
fú líng	poria
gān cǎo	baked licorice [root]
pào jiāng	blast-fried ginger
bò hé	mint

This prescription primarily treats liver depression and blood vacuity with intermittent fever and chills, headache, costal pain, anorexia, irregular menstruation, and a wiry vacuity pulse. Nonetheless, it does not purely soothe the liver but is also used to strengthen the spleen. Therefore, *dāng guī* (tangkuei) and *bái sháo yào* (white peony [root]) are used in the prescription to nourish the liver, *chái hú* (bupleurum [root]) courses the liver to promote orderly extension, *cāng zhú* (atractylodes [root]), *fú líng* (poria), and *gān cǎo* (licorice [root]) shore up the middle and prevent spleen-earth from being overly restrained by wood. A little of both *bò hé* (mint) and *pào jiāng* (blast-fried ginger) are used in the decoction because they also assist the capacity of the prescription to soothe depression and harmonize the middle. Later practitioners added *mǔ dān pí* (moutan [root bark]) and *shān zhī zǐ* (gardenia [fruit]) to treat depressive liver with an effulgence of fire to yield *Jiā Wèi Xiāo Yáo Sǎn* (Supplemented Free Wanderer Powder). Raw or cooked *dì huáng* (rehmannia [root]) is added in the case of blood vacuity to yield *Hēi Xiāo Yáo Sǎn* (Black Free Wanderer Powder), although the orientation of the therapy remains the same. Because *Xiāo Yán Sǎn* (Free Wanderer Powder) courses the liver and strengthens the spleen, it has generally come to be explained as treating an effulgence of wood overly restraining earth. My view is that an effulgence of wood restraining earth implies that the liver is strong and the spleen is weak. However, Free Wanderer Powder primarily treats a dual vacuity of liver and spleen, or wood not coursing earth. The liver is consequently incapable of being coursed, drained, and disinhibited, and the spleen is also unable to strengthen [i.e., effectively govern] transportation and generate transformation. They both become encumbered and depressive symptoms occur. Nourishing the liver and soothing the qi, and supplementing the spleen and harmonizing the middle are all accomplished based on the fundamental principle, "If there is a depression of wood, resolve it." For instance, the strength of *dāng guī* (tangkuei), *bái sháo yào* (white peony [root]), and *chái hú* (bupleurum [root]), which are used in the case of liver effulgence, only support the qi fire. If the spleen is excessively restrained, *cāng zhú* (atractylodes [root]), *gān cǎo* (licorice [root]), and *fú líng* (poria) will only promote stasis.

Vacuity and repletion must be clearly discriminated and we must understand that the root symptom of intermittent fever and chills is not the same as the similar *shào yáng* pattern. Headache and costal distension are not the same as horizontal counterflow of liver qi, and a diminished appetite is not the same as repletion fullness in the stomach. Therefore, this prescription cannot be simplistically used as the primary prescription for coursing the liver.

Translator's Comment

The precision involved in differentiating between wood not restraining earth and wood restraining earth pathologically is characteristic of Qin Bowei's approach to Chinese medicine. These two patterns, although distinct, have such an overall similarity that careful examination is required to discriminate between them in the clinic. The following is a summary of how Qin Bowei discriminates these two patterns.

Wood not restraining earth is characterized by a depression of liver qi, which is then incapable of coursing the stomach and spleen. Clinically, however, the emphasis is on the earth phase and there is a predominance of symptoms involving stagnation within the stomach. These symptoms include thoracic oppression, nausea, slow digestion, and abdominal distension. Therapeutically, earth is often harmonized with damp-transforming stomach- and spleen-regulating medicinals. When this is accomplished, the liver becomes regulated without further intervention. Examples of this approach include *Jiě Gān Qiān* (Liver-Resolving Brew) and *Wēn Dǎn Tāng* (Gallbladder-Warming Decoction). Nonetheless, there are also therapeutic approaches that directly course the liver while regulating earth. Qin Bowei cites *chái hú* (bupleurum [root]) as the primary medicinal for coursing the liver in cases of wood not retraining earth. His interpretation of *Xiāo Yáo Sǎn* (Free Wanderer Powder) as a medicinal formula addressing a dual liver and spleen vacuity and wood failing to course earth is another clear example of this approach.

Wood overly restraining earth is characterized by a depression of qi that has counterflowed, impairing the stomach and spleen. In general, the emphasis is on liver wood and thus calls for treatment methods for coursing and draining the liver while regulating the stomach and spleen. Qin Bowei cites *Yì Mù Hé Zhōng Tāng* (Wood-Repressing Center-Harmonizing Decoction) as an example of this approach. *Qīng pí* (unripe tangerine peel) and *xiāng fù zǐ* (cyperus [root]) are cited as the primary medicinals used in the case of wood overly restraining earth. Qin Bowei's discussion of *Tòng Xiè Yào Fāng* (Pain and Diarrhea Formula) is evidence that coursing and draining is not the only therapeutic approach that can be taken. *Bái sháo yào* (white peony [root]) is used in this prescription not to course the liver but to constrain it. The idea is that if the liver were to nourish the effulgence within, it would harmonize on its own.

The value of such distinctions may not be readily apparent in general descriptions of a clinical landscape because the major features are all the same. On the other hand, these discriminations are essential to fine-tuning the selection of prescriptions and their component medicinals.

Dān Shēn Yǐn (Salvia Beverage)	
from *Yī Xué Jīn Zhēn*	
dān shēn	salvia [root]
tán xiāng	sandalwood
shā rén	amomum [fruit]

While this prescription was used originally to treat cardiac and gastric pain from qi stasis and depressive binding, I also use it to good effect for costal pain in the network vessels that is influencing the intestines and stomach. *Dān shēn* (salvia [root]) is chosen to harmonize the blood, *tán xiāng* (sandalwood) to regulate the qi, and *bái dòu kòu* (cardamom) to harmonize the middle. If the pain is intense, then *yù jīn* (curcuma [tuber]) and *rǔ xiāng* (frankincense) may be combined with this prescription.

Yī Guàn Jiān (All-the-Way-Through Brew)	
from *Liǔ Jōu Yī Huò*	
běi shā shēn	glehnia [root]
mài mén dōng	ophiopogon [tuber]
dāng guī	tangkuei
xiān dì huáng	fresh rehmannia [root]
chuān liàn zǐ	toosendan [fruit]

While the treatment of liver qi is not generally difficult, it is difficult to treat an insufficiency of liver yin occuring together with a horizontal counterflow of liver qi. We are encumbered by the fact that a great many medicinals for regulating the qi and coursing the liver are fragrant and drying and injure the yin, and in this lies an essential contradiction.[43] [In

---

[43]Trans: The contradiction here is in the intent. Qi regulating medicinals dry the yin but medicinals that moisten the yin promote qi stasis.

this prescription] the medicinals for enriching the liver and moistening dryness are asssisted by a small amount of *chuān liàn zǐ* (toosendan [fruit]). Nourishing the liver viscus soothes the liver. Thus a liver vacuity qi stasis, which gives rise to symptoms such as thoracocostal fullness and pain, acid regurgitation, a bitter taste in the mouth, shan qi, and accumulations and conglomerations may be relaxed and resolved. This is said to be a method outside the scope of other methods.

Methods of modification are pointed out in *Liǔ Zhōu Yī Huò*. For instance, to treat binding constipation, add *guā lóu zǐ* (trichosanthes seed). For vacuity heat causing copious perspiration, add *dì gǔ pí* (lycium root bark). For copious phlegm, add *bèi mǔ* (fritillaria [bulb]). For a dry red tongue, add *shí hú* (dendrobium [stem]). For abdominal pain, add *bái sháo yào* (white peony [root]) and *gān cǎo* (licorice [root]). For costal pain and distension where a hard lump may be palpated, add *biē jiǎ* (turtle shell).

Lóng Dǎn Xiè Gān Tāng (Gentian Liver-Draining Decoction)	
from *Hé Jì Jú Fāng*	
lóng dǎn	gentian [root]
huáng qín	scutellaria [root]
shān zhī zǐ	gardenia [fruit]
zé xiè	alisma [tuber]
mù tōng	mutong [stem]
chē qián zǐ	plantago seed
dāng guī	tangkuei
chái hú	bupleurum [root]
xiān dì huáng	raw rehmannia [root]
gān cǎo	licorice [root]

Lóng dǎn (gentian [root]) is the sovereign in this prescription, and when combined with *huáng qín* (scutellaria [root]), and *shān zhī zǐ* (gardenia [fruit]), it drains repletion fire from the liver and gallbladder. *Mù tōng* (mutong [stem]), *chē qián zǐ* (plantago seed), and *zé xiè* alisma [tuber]) clear heat and disinhibit dampness. *Xiān dì huáng* (fresh rehmannia [root]) and *dāng guī* (tangkuei) are employed to protect the overflow of fire from injuring the yin. *Gān cǎo* (licorice [root]) is used to harmonize the middle and resolve toxins, and *chái hú* (bupleurum [root]) is used to guide the channels and course the qi. In general, the [prescription] functions via the direct use of bitter cold medicinals, which act to drain liver fire and to clear and disinhibit damp-heat from the lower burner. This formula therefore treats symptoms such as costal pain, bitter taste in the mouth, red eyes, and tinnitus from an upward counterflow of liver fire, as well as symptoms of dribbling urination, genital swelling, and itching, all from dampness and heat pouring downward.

Dāng Guī Lóng Huì Wán (Tangkuei, Gentian, and Aloe Pill)	
from *Xuān Míng Lǔn Fāng*	
dāng guī	tangkuei
lóng dǎn	gentian [root]
lú gēn	phragmites [root]

huáng lián	coptis [root]
huáng bǎi	phellodendron [bark]
dà huáng	rhubarb
huáng qín	scutellaria [root]
shān zhī zǐ	gardenia [fruit]
qīng dài	indigo
mù xiāng	saussurea [root]
shè xiāng	musk

This prescription drains repletion fire from the liver channel and is based on a foundation of *Huáng Lián Jiě Dú Tāng* (Coptis Toxin-Resolving Decoction) [to which] is added *dà huáng* (rhubarb) and *lú gēn* (phragmites [root]). The strength of this bitter cold, fire draining prescription outstrips that of *Lóng Dǎn Xiè Gān Tāng,* and moreover it frees and disinhibits the stools. Also, the use of *qīng dài* (indigo), *mù xiang* (saussurea [root]), and *shè xiāng* (musk) clears the constructive and resolves toxins, regulates the qi, and tracks wind. This prescription is also specific for a surging of liver fire causing unconsciousness, with the development of symptoms of delirium, fright palpitations, and twitching.

Xiè Qīng Wán (Green-Blue Draining Pills)	
from *Xiǎo Ér Yào Zhèng Zhí Jué*	
dāng guī	tangkuei
lóng dǎn	gentian [root]
shān zhī zǐ	gardenia [fruit]
dà huáng	rhubarb
chuān xiōng	ligusticum [root]
qiāng huó	notopterygium [root]
fáng fēng	ledebouriella [root]

This prescription primarily treats vexation, agitation, and insomnia from liver fire, with symptoms of a tendency to be easily frightened, frequent anger, and red eyes that are swollen and painful. The prescription employs *lóng dǎn* (gentian [root]), *shān zhī zǐ* (gardenia [fruit]), and *dà huáng* (rhubarb) as bitter cold medicinals for draining heat. *Dāng guī* (tangkuei), *chuān xiōng* (ligusticum [root]), *qiāng huó* (notopterygium [root]), and *fáng fēng* (ledebouriella [root]) nourish the blood and track wind, and are able to simultaneously dissipate depressive fire.

It should be noted that *Xiè Qīng Wán* (Green-Blue Draining Pill), *Lóng Dǎn Xiè Gān [Tāng]* (Gentian Liver-Draining Decoction), and *Dāng Guī Lóng Huì Wán* (Tangkuei, Gentian, and Aloe Pill) are all used for repletion fire. All of these prescriptions use bitter cold methods for directly breaking repletion fire. *Dāng Guī Lóng Huì [Wán]* is the strongest [prescription] for draining fire, followed by *Lóng Dǎn Xiè Gān [Tāng],* and *Xiè Qīng [Wán],* each being relatively milder. The three prescriptions are distinct, with *Lóng Dǎn Xiè Gān [Tāng]* simultaneously disinhibiting urination, *Dāng Guī Lóng Huì [Wán]* able to free the stools, and *Xiè Qīng [Wán]* being used to track wind and dissipate fire rather than to free elimination.

Dāng Guī Sì Nì Tāng (Tangkuei Counterflow Cold Decoction)	
from the *Shāng Hán Lùn*	
dāng guī	tangkuei
guì zhī	cinnamon twig
bái sháo yào	white peony [root]
xì xīn	asarum
gān cǎo	baked licorice [root]
tōng cǎo	rice-paper plant pith
suān zǎo rén	spiny jujube [kernel]

This prescription primarily treats cold damage to the *jué yīn* liver,[44] with counterflow cold [in the] extremities and a fine pulse verging on expiry. Furthermore, this prescription is related to prescriptions for warming the liver, dispelling cold, and nourishing the blood vessels. In the case of longstanding cold, *wú zhū yú* (evodia [fruit]) and *shēng jiāng* (fresh ginger) may be added. This prescription is then called *Dāng Guī Sì Nì Wú Zhū Yú Shēng Jiāng Tāng* (Tangkuei Counterflow Cold Decoction Plus Evodia and Fresh Ginger).

In general, when the liver viscera contracts cold or there is a complete vacuity within the entire body, this prescription – or a modified version of this presecription – becomes the primary prescription for warming the liver. In using warming methods to treating liver illnesses, regardless of the presence of cold and the necessity for the retrieval of yang, *guì zhī* (cinnamon twig), *xì xīn* (asarum), *wú zhū yú* (evodia [fruit]), and *chuān liàn zǐ* (toosendan [fruit]) are to be used rather than *fù zǐ* (aconite [accessory tuber]), and *gān jiāng* (dried ginger [root]). Furthermore, where there are many vacuity symptoms *ròu guì* (cinnamon bark) may be used because it enters the blood portion of the liver and assists the production of qi.

Chén Píngpó once advanced his doubts regarding this prescription:

> *Why is it that in treating four counterflows Zhòng Jǐng employed gān jiāng (dried ginger [root]) and chuān wū tóu (aconite main tuber)? In the base prescription there are no medicinals from the categories of warming the middle and assisting the yang, yet in longstanding cold wú zhū yu (evodia [fruit]) and shēng jiāng (fresh ginger) are nevertheless added instead of gān jiāng (dried ginger) or fù zǐ (aconite [accessory tuber]).*

I think he has some insight here. Nonetheless, also insufficient is his explanation:[45]

> *The jué yīn liver viscera stores the ying blood and is wood. Gall-bladder fire depends upon it internally, wind and fire have the same source. If one is not suffering from pathogenic cold and internal imbalance, and if yang's generation of qi verges on expiry, then materials that are acrid and warm should not be used, lest this harass wind fire into mobility.*

---

[44]Trans: The expression *"jué yīn* liver" here, in distinction to Qin's "liver viscus," implies some degree of channel involvement expressed as cold extremities.

[45]Trans: This is not clear; neither, however is the Chinese, nor does Qin provide any further explanation.

Nuǎn Gān Jiān (Liver-Warming Brew)	
from *Jǐng Yuè Quán Shū*	
dāng guī	tangkuei
gǒu qǐ zǐ	lycium [berry]
xiǎo huí xiāng	fennel [fruit]
ròu guì	cinnamon bark
wū yào	lindera [root]
chén xiāng	aquilaria [wood]
fú líng	poria

While this prescription is primarily for warming the liver, it is simultaneously used to move the qi, dissipate cold, and disinhibit dampness in the treatment of the symptoms of lower abdominal pain and soreness and shan qi. It is organized so that *dāng guī* (tangkuei) and *gǒu qǐ zǐ* (lycium [berry]) warm and supplement the liver viscus, *ròu guì* (cinnamon bark) and *hú lú bā* (foenugreek [seed]) warm the channels and dissipate cold, *wū yào* (lindera [root]) and *chén xiāng* (aquilaria [wood]) free and rectify the qi, and *fú líng* (poria) disinhibits dampness and frees the yang. Whenever there is liver cold qi stasis, and the symptoms tend to be focused in the lower burner, a modified form of this prescription can be used.

Wū Méi Wán (Mume Pill)	
from *Shāng Hán Lùn*	
wū méi	mume [fruit]
dāng guī	tangkuei
guì zhī	cinnamon twig
xì xīn	asarum
shǔ jiāo	zanthoxylum [husk]
gān jiāng	dried ginger [root]
fù zǐ	aconite [accessory tuber]
rén shēn	ginseng
huáng lián	coptis [root]
huáng bǎi	phellodendron [bark]

This prescription treats vacuity weakness of the correct qi of the liver viscus and symptoms of mixed chills and fever. It uses *rén shēn* (ginseng), and *dāng guī* (tangkuei), to supplement the qi and blood, *xì xīn* (asarum), *gān jiāng* (dried ginger [root]), *fù zǐ* (aconite [accessory tuber]), *guì zhī* (cinnamon twig), and *shǔ jiāo* (zanthoxylum [husk]) to warm cold and free the blood vessels, while *huáng lián* (coptis [root]) and *huáng bǎi* (phellodendron [bark]) clear fire. In addition, the sour taste of *wū méi* (mume [fruit]) enters the liver as the sovereign, the combined strength of the assisting medicinals entering a single channel. It is able to treat symptoms of abdominal pain, vomiting, dysentery, and roundworm reversal. Nonetheless, the overall nature of the prescription tends to be warming, and it is thus indicated for severe cold conditions.

Qīng Hào Biē Jiǎ Tāng (Sweet Wormwood and Turtle Shell Decoction)	
from Wēn Bìng Tiáo Biàn	
yīn chén hāo	capillaris
biē jiǎ	turtle shell
xiān dì huáng	raw fresh rehmannia [root]
zhī mǔ	anemarrhena [root]
mǔ dān pí	moutan [root bark]

This prescription was originally used to treat pathogens from thermic disease hidden in the yin aspect, as well as tidal fever from liver vacuity. *Biē jiǎ* (turtle shell) enters the liver and enriches the yin, and *mǔ dān pí* (moutan [root bark]) cools the liver. *Yīn chén hāo* (capillaris) clears and evicts heat from the *shào yáng*. These medicinals are assisted by *xiān dì huáng* (fresh rehmannia [root]) and *zhī mǔ* (anemarrhena [root]), which nourish the yin and abate steaming. These medicinals are precisely balanced to address a liver vacuity presenting as tidal fever. Such a tidal fever most often develops in the afternoon and is accompanied by perspiration with fatigue. The [patient's] body is emaciated and the pulse is fine, weak, and rapid.

Biē Jiǎ Jiān Wán (Turtle Shell Decocted Pill)	
from Jīn Guì Yào Luè	
biē jiǎ	turtle shell
wū shàn	belamcanda [root]
huáng qín	scutellaria [root]
chái hú	bupleurum [root]
shǔ fù	wood louse
gān jiāng	dried ginger
dà huáng	rhubarb
bái sháo yào	white peony [root]
guì zhī	cinnamon twig
zǐ wēi gēn	campsis [root]
shí wéi	pyrrosia [leaf]
hòu pò	magnolia bark
mǔ dān pí	moutan [root bark]
qū mài	dianthus
tíng lì zǐ	tingli [seed]
bàn xià	pinellia [tuber]
rén shēn	ginseng
zhè chóng	wingless cockroach
ē jiāo	ass hide glue
lù fāng fáng	hornet's nest
xiáo shí	niter
xiáng láng	dung beetle
táo rén	peach kernel

This prescription was originally used to treat malarial lump glomus.[46]

---

[46]A localized subjective feeling of fullness and blockage in the chest. In severe cases it can be associated with a feeling of oppression. In the abdomen, glomus is the sensation of a lump that cannot be detected by palpation.

Turtle shell is the sovereign, and functions to soften hardness and dissipating bondage. It enters the liver and tracks down pathogens. In later times, this formula has been used for glomus lumps due to liver accumulation. The prescription predominately contains medicinals that disinhibit the qi, dissipate water, and move blood stasis, with the intent of dissipating binding stasis. Although the prescription contains *rén shēn* (ginseng) and *ē jiāo* (ass hide glue) to supplement the qi and nourish the blood, these [ingredients] are unable to withstand and counteract the strength of the other dissipating medicinals.[47] Therefore, when this prescription is administered, the patient will often report a feeling of fatigue. As a result it is contraindicated in vacuity conditions and this prescription should not be administered over an extended period, even to strong patients.

Zuǒ Jīn Wǎn (Left-Running Metal Pill)	
from *Dān Xī Xīn Fǎ*	
huáng lián	coptis [root]
wú zhū yú	evodia [fruit]

This prescription primarily treats costal pain due to liver fire, presenting with acid regurgitation and gastric upset, bitter taste in the mouth, red tongue, and wiry rapid pulse. Because *huáng lián* (coptis [root]) enters the heart while *wú zhū yú* (evodia [fruit]) enters the liver, and the dose of *huáng lián* (coptis [root]) is six times that of *wú zhū yú*, the prescription can therefore be explained primarily in terms of actually draining repletion from the son, making evodia the assisting medicinal. I know that warming medicinals are very rarely used as assistants in liver fire conditions. However, *huáng lián* (coptis [root]) and *wú zhū yú* (evodia [fruit]) function in a unique manner, and it is difficult to explain [their functions only in relation to their thermic qualities]. In researching the effects of this prescription, it is clear that the acid regurgitation and gastric upset are the most pronounced symptoms and the main effect of this prescription is on the stomach. *Huáng lián* is capable of bitter downbearing and harmonization of the stomach. *Wú zhū yú* also dissipates binding depression of the stomach qi, and these two are used together in the acrid bitter category of [medicinals in] *Xiè Xīn Tāng* (Heart-Draining Decoction). Therefore, in cases of acid regurgitation with simultaneous phlegm dampness and thick snivel, the dosage of *wú zhū yú* (evodia [fruit]), may be increased for the best result.

Liáng Fù Wán (Lesser Galangal and Cyperus Pill)	
from *Liáng Fāng Jí Yòng*	
gāo liáng jiāng	lesser galangal root
xiāng fù zǐ	cyperus [root]

This prescription is effective in the treatment of liver and stomach qi pain which tends to be cold in nature. As to the functions of these two medicinals, *gāo liáng jiāng* (lesser galangal [root]) warms the stomach and dissipates cold, while *xiāng fù zǐ* (cyperus [root]) courses the liver and circulates the qi. Generally the dose of both medicinals is equal and they mutually support one another. Nonetheless, if cold predominates in the clinical picture then the dose of *gāo liáng jiāng* is doubled, while, if qi [stasis] predominates, the dose of *xiāng fù zǐ* is doubled.

---

[47]Trans: The prescription attacks the pathogen much more strongly than it supports the qi and is thus heavily weighted toward dissipation.

Jīn Líng Zǐ Sàn (Toosendan Powder)

from *Shèng Huì Fāng*

chuān liàn zǐ	toosendan [fruit]
xuán hú suǒ	corydalis [tuber]

This prescription primarily treats depressive stasis from liver qi and liver fire, with symptoms of costal pain and lower abdominal distension and pain. The prescription contains only two medicinals and they are in equal doses. As it is named after *chuān liàn zǐ* (toosendan [fruit]), it is clear that the prescription's predominant funtions are those of coursing the qi and draining liver fire. Toosendan enters the qi aspect and also tends to be bitter and cold. Combined with the acrid and warm blood vitalizing corydalis, it moves the qi and arrests pain.

Sì Mó Yǐn (Four Milled Ingredients Beverage)

from *Jì Shēng Fāng*

chén xiāng	aquilaria [wood]
tài wū yào	lindera [root]
bīn láng	areca [nut]
rén shēn	ginseng

This prescription treats horizontal counterflow of liver qi that is upwardly attacking the lung viscus, or attacking horizontally to the spleen-stomach.[48] This precipitates an ascent of qi with the consequences of panting respiration, thoracic fullness and anorexia, and in extreme cases clouding reversal.[49]

Chén xiāng (aquilaria [wood]) is the primary medicinal, *bīn láng* (areca [nut]), and *wū yào* (lindera [root]) are guides, downbearing and circulating the qi, so the thrust of the prescription is [thus] focused in a single direction. Ginseng is used lest the other medicinals harm and dissipate the correct qi. If *rén shēn* (ginseng) is deleted, then *mù xiāng* (saussurea [root]) and *zhǐ ké* (bitter orange) are to be added, resulting in the prescription known as *Wǔ Mó Yǐn Zǐ* (Five Milled Ingredients Drink), thus becoming a simple qi-regulating prescription.

Bái Zhú Sháo Yào Sǎn (Ovate Atractylodes and Peony Powder)

from *Luí Cǎo Cuān Fāng*

bái zhú	ovate atractylodes [root]
bái sháo yào	white peony [root]
chén pí	tangerine peel
fáng fēng	ledebouriella [root]

This prescription is also called *Tòng Xiè Yào Fāng* (Pain and Diarrhea Formula) and primarily treats diarrhea that occurs with liver effulgence and spleen weakness, as well as occasional diarrhea, with abdominal pain and borborygmus. Because there is liver effulgence and spleen weakness, *bái sháo yào* (white peony [root]) is used to restrain the liver and *cāng zhú* (atractylodes [root]) is used to strengthen the spleen. Because there is indigestion and severe intra-abdominal qi distension [associated with this

---

[48]Qin Bowei clearly includes a counterflow of liver qi into the lung as well as the more familiar invasion of the stomach and spleen in his definition of horizontal counterflow.

[49]Sudden loss of consciousness, sometimes accompanied by reversal frigidity of the limbs. It differs from clouded spirit (or clouding of the spirit) in that it is of short duration.

pattern], these medicinals are therefore assisted by *chén pí* (tangerine peel) to regulate the qi and harmonize the middle, as well as *fáng fēng* (ledebouriella [root]) to regulate the liver and soothe the spleen to dissipate qi stasis. Diarrhea from liver effulgence and spleen weakness will most often be preceded by distension and then pain. The diarrhea will not be copious and the symptoms will be relieved following the diarrhea. This pattern will be repeated. The pulse is typically wiry and fine, the right being more exuberant than the left. These manifestations reflect the condition of wood overwhelming earth. If the tongue body is red and seamed, with a yellow dry or slimy moss, with thirst and vexation oppression, irritability and sensation of pressure in the head, rough voidings of dark urine, and anal burning following diarrhea, then *tǔ huò xiāng* (agastache), *huáng lián* (coptis [root]), *gé gēn* (pueraria [root]), and *méi huā* (mume flower) may be added.

Wēn Dǎn Tāng (Gallbladder-Warming Decoction)	
from *Qiān Jīn Fāng*	
chén pí	tangerine peel
bàn xià	pinellia [tuber]
fú líng	poria
zhǐ shí	unripe bitter orange
gān cǎo	licorice [root]
zhú rú	bamboo shavings

The intent of this prescription is to harmonize the stomach, transform phlegm and clear heat, so it is not a prescription that [primarily] addresses liver illnesses. Because the gallbladder is attached to the liver, its nature is warm, and it governs the upbearing of the qi, if there is depressive stasis of the liver qi, then the gallbladder qi is not soothed, and it cannot course earth. This presents as gastric symptoms such as thoracic oppression and nausea. If the counterflow of stomach qi is healed, then the depression of gallbladder qi will also be healed. Therefore one should harmonize and downbear the stomach qi to treat the branch. This indirectly soothes and unfolds the gallbladder qi, and therefore the liver qi also becomes relaxed and harmonized. The reference to "warming the gallbladder" in regard to this prescription is based on the quality of the gallbladder that functions to upbear the qi. [Therefore,] the meaning of the word "warming" in this context is completely different from the [meaning of the] warming characters used for [the concepts of] warming the spleen or warming the kidney.

Enumerated above are the prescriptions commonly used in liver illnesses. Some are prescriptions [specifically designed] for liver illnesses and some are not, and among the prescriptions for liver illnesses, many are modified in treatment. This clarifies the range of prescriptions that treat liver illnesses and demonstrates that they are principally selected for use based not only on etiology and pathomechanism but also on the symptoms presented by the illness.

If we assume that only prescriptions specifically designed for liver illnesses must be selected to treat liver illnesses, or [if we] assume that a prescription for a particular liver illness in fact treats only a liver illness, then the available avenues for the treatment of liver illnesses are extremely narrow. To truly grasp these prescriptions, we must understand the agility with which they are to be used, and modify them skillfully.

Yī Chún Téng Yì contains a large number of prescriptions composed specifically for liver illnesses, and some that are closely related to liver illness [prescriptions], and these also merit investigation. [We discuss these in the following sections.]

Yì Mù Hé Zhōng Tāng	
WOOD REPRESSING CENTER-HARMONIZING DECOCTION	
dāng guī	tangkuei
qīng pí	unripe tangerine peel
cì jí lí	tribulus [fruit]
chén pí	tangerine peel
yù jīn	curcuma [tuber]
cāng zhú	atractylodes [root]
bái zhú	ovate atractylodes [root]
hòu pò	magnolia bark
mù xiāng	saussurea [root]
shā rén	amomum [fruit]
fú líng	poria
fó gān	Buddha's hand [fruit]
tán xiāng	sandalwood

This prescription is indicated for excessive strength of liver qi, which overly restrains the spleen and stomach. The middle cavity is not soothed and there is diminished appetite.[50] The left *guān* pulse is extremely wiry and there is a deep fine quality to the right position.

Zī Shēng Qīng Yǎng Tāng	
ENRICHING AND ENGENDERING YANG-CLEARING DECOCTION	
dì huáng	rehmannia [root]
bái sháo yào	white peony [root]
mài mén dōng	ophiopogon [tuber]
shí hú	dendrobium [stem]
jú huā	chrysanthemum [flower]
sāng yè	mulberry leaf
mǔ dān pí	moutan [root bark]
shí jué míng	abalone shell
cí shí	loadstone
tiān má	gastrodia [root]
bò hé	mint
chái hú	bupleurum [root]

This prescription is indicated for liver wind, cephalic and visual dizziness, spasmodic joints and twitching, and a feeling as if ascending through clouds and mist or like sitting in a boat.

---

[50]Trans: Qin Bowei refers here to the "Central Venter," thus making reference to the acupoint CV-12.

Zhū Yú Fù Guì Tāng	
EVODIA, ACONITE, AND CINNAMON BARK DECOCTION	
wú zhū yú	evodia [fruit]
fù zǐ	aconite [accessory tuber]
ròu guì	cinnamon bark
dāng guī	tangkuei
bái sháo yào	white peony [root]
bái zhú	ovate atractylodes [root]
wū yào	lindera [root]
suān zǎo rén	spiny jujube [kernel]

This prescription is indicated for pathogenic cold that directly enters the liver channel, with symptoms of gripping pain in the subcostal and abdominal regions, dysentery, reversal chill of the hands and foot, and a green-blue color to the fingernails.

Hán Mù Yǎng Yíng Tāng	
WOOD-MOISTENING CONSTRUCTION-NOURISHING DECOCTION	
dì huáng	rehmannia [root]
rén shēn	ginseng
mài mén dōng	ophiopogon [tuber]
dà zǎo	jujube
wǔ wèi zǐ	schisandra [berry]
dāng guī	tangkuei
bái sháo yào	white peony [root]
suān zǎo rén	spiny jujube [kernel]
qín jiāo	large gentian [root]
mù guā	chaenomeles [fruit]

This prescription is indicated for contraction of dry heat by the liver, with dessication and withering of the blood aspect, sinew contraction, and withering.

Jiā Wèi Dān Zhī Zǐ Tāng	
SUPPLEMENTED MOUTAN AND GARDENIA DECOCTION	
mǔ dān pí	moutan [root bark]
shān zhī zǐ	gardenia [fruit]
dì huáng	rehmannia [root]
chì sháo yào	red peony [root]
lóng dǎn	gentian [root]
xià kū cǎo	prunella [spike]
mù tōng	mutong [stem]
chē qián zǐ	plantago seed
chái hú	bupleurum [root]
tōng cǎo	rice-paper plant pith

This prescription is indicated for exuberance of fire in the liver-gallbladder with costal pain, deafness, bitter taste in the mouth, sinew atony, genital pain and turbid strangury, and hematuria.

Jiě Yù Hé Huān Tāng
DEPRESSION-RESOLVING ALBIZZIA DECOCTION

hé huān huā	silk tree flower
yù jīn	curcuma [tuber]
dāng guī	tangkuei
chén xiāng	aquilaria [wood]
bái sháo yào	white peony [root]
dān shēn	salvia [root]
shān zhī zǐ	gardenia [fruit]
bǎi zǐ rén	biota seed
fú líng	poria
chái hú	bupleurum [root]
bò hé	mint
dà zǎo	jujube

This prescription is indicated for depression due to unfulfilled aspirations, extreme depression of qi generating fire, cardiac vexation and worry, fever, and irritability.

Guī Guī Huà Nì Tāng
ANGELICA AND CINNAMON COUNTERFLOW TRANSFORMING DECOCTION

dāng guī	tangkuei
bái sháo yào	white peony [root]
guì zhī	cinnamon twig
qīng pí	unripe tangerine peel
cì jí lí	tribulus [fruit]
yù jīn	curcuma [tuber]
hé huān huā	silk tree flower
méi guī huā	rose
fú líng	poria
mù xiāng	saussurea [root]
tǔ niú xī	native achyranthes [root]
jiàng zhēn xiāng	dalbergia [wood]
dà zǎo	jujube

This prescription is indicated for blood vacuity and hindrance from depressive binding of liver qi.

Dān Qīng Yǐn
ELIXIR CLEARING DRINK

dài zhě shí	hematite
qīng dài	indigo

mixed with:

mài mén dōng	ophiopogon [tuber]
běi shā shēn	glehnia [root]
shí hú	dendrobium [stem]
bèi mǔ	fritillaria [bulb]
xìng rén	apricot kernel
cì jí lí	tribulus [fruit]
jú huā	chrysanthemum [flower]
sāng yè	mulberry leaf

This prescription is indicated for liver fire attacking the lung, cough with scanty phlegm, costal pain, tendency to become easily angered, and cephalic dizziness.

Qīng Yáng Tāng	
YANG CLEARING DECOCTION	
qīng chén pí	unripe and ripe tangerine peel
chái hú	bupleurum [root]
cì jí lí	tribulus [fruit]
yù jīn	curcuma [tuber]
yán hú suǒ	corydalis [tuber]
wū yào	lindera [root]
mù xiāng	saussurea [root]
pào jiāng	blast-fried ginger
shǔ jiāo	zanthoxylum [husk]

This prescription is indicated for liver cold qi stasis, subcostal distension and fullness, and a drawing pain in the lower abdomen.

Fú Yáng Guī Huà Tāng	
YANG SUPPORTING RETURNING AND TRANSFORMING DECOCTION	
dǎng shēn	codonopsis [root]
fú líng	poria
bái zhú	ovate atractylodes [root]
hòu pò	magnolia bark
shā rén	amomum [fruit]
fù zǐ	aconite [accessory tuber]
dāng guī	tangkuei
qīng chén pí	ripe and unripe tangerine peel
cì jí lí	tribulus [fruit]
mù guā	chaenomeles [fruit]
niú xī	achyranthes [root]
chē qián zǐ	plantago seed
gān jiāng	dried ginger [root]

This prescription is indicated for drum distension and the presence of green-blue veins on the abdomen, from an effulgence of wood overwhelming earth.

Líng Yáng Jiǎo Tāng	
ANTELOPE HORN DECOCTION	
líng yáng jiǎo	antelope horn
guī bǎn	tortoise plastron
xiān dì huáng	fresh rehmannia [root]
bái sháo yào	white peony [root]
mǔ dān pí	moutan [root bark]
jú huā	chrysanthemum [flower]
xià kū cǎo	prunella [spike]
shí jué míng	abalone shell
chán tuì	cicada molting
bò hé	mint
dà zǎo	jujube

This [prescription] is indicated for a stirring of liver heat and ascension of liver yang with a splitting headache, contracture of the sinew vessels,[51] and pain that connects to the eyeball.

Yǎng Xuě Shèng Fēng Tāng	
BLOOD-NOURISHING WIND-OVERCOMING DECOCTION	
dì huáng	rehmannia [root]
dāng guī	tangkuei
bái sháo yào	white peony [root]
chuān xiōng	ligusticum [root]
gǒu qǐ zǐ	lycium [berry]
wǔ wèi zǐ	schisandra [berry]
jú huā	chrysanthemum [flower]
sāng yè	mulberry leaf
zhī má	sesame [seed]
dà zǎo	jujube

This prescription is indicated for headache from vacuity of liver blood, a subjective sensation of emptiness in the head and brain, visual dullness, and dizziness.[52]

Tiáo Yíng Liàn Gān Yǐn	
CONSTRUCTION-REGULATING LIVER-CONSTRAINING DRINK	
dāng guī	tangkuei
bái sháo yào	white peony [root]
ē jiāo	ass hide glue
gǒu qǐ zǐ	lycium [berry]
chuān xiōng	ligusticum [root]
wǔ wèi zǐ	schisandra [berry]
suān zǎo rén	spiny jujube [kernel]
fú líng	poria
chén pí	tangerine peel
mù xiāng	saussurea [root]
gān jiāng	dried ginger [root]
dà zǎo	jujube

This prescription is indicated for vacuity of liver blood, qi counterflow, and distension and pain in the stomach cavity.

All these prescriptions have been developed from experience in clinical practice. We can see how they treat the primary symptoms, how they treat associated symptoms, how they relate to the viscera, and how the base prescriptions can be modified. They prove very inspiring in clinical practice.

---

[51]Permanent contraction or hypertension of the musculature.

[52]Visual dizziness, *xuàn:* Clouded flowery vision; often associated with mental dizziness.

It must be added that the organization of prescriptions, their therapeutic effects, and their relative doses are intimately related. In these prescriptions the doses of the medicinals for enriching and supplementing the liver and kidney are relatively heavy. The doses of medicinals for restraining and calming are also heavy. The doses of medicinals for regulating the qi, harmonizing the blood, clearing heat, and descending fire tend to be the standard doses used for those [medicinals] in general. For instance, if *chái hú* (bupleurum [root]) and *bò hé* (mint) are used to diffuse and dissipate depressive fire, the doses should typically not exceed one *qián*.

Discrimination of Prescriptions

Prescription	Pattern	Guiding Symptoms
Sì Wù Tāng	Vacuity of liver blood	
Zī Shuǐ Qīng Gān Yǐn	Vacuity of liver blood accompanied by depressive fire	Remittent fever, intercostal qi stasis, vomiting of sour fluid
Líng Yáng Gōu Téng Tāng	Pathogenic heat in *jué yīn*	Clouding of the spirit and convulsion
Dà Dìng Fēng Zhū Tàng	Pathogenic heat dissipating the true yin	Lassitude
Zhēn Zhū Mǔ Wán	Insufficiency of liver blood and wind yang	Dizziness, flowery vision, and restless sleep
Sǎng Má Wǎn	Vacuity of liver and kidney with blood heat and wind yang	Liver yang headache and dizziness
Xiǎo Chái Hú Tāng	Pathogenic cold in the *shào yáng*	Intermittent chills and fever, thoracocostal fullness, vexation and nausea
Sì Nì Sǎn	Transmission of pathogenic heat due to qi depression	Cold extremities, gastric distress
Chái Hǔ Shū Gān Sǎn	Disharmony of qi and blood	Costal pain and fever and chills
Jiě Gān Qiān	Qi stasis causing dampness and disharmony of the middle qi	Impaired digestion and abdominal distension
Huà Gān Qiān	Internal depression of fire qi in the liver causing upward counterflow	Bloody phlegmatic cough
Yuè Jú Wán	Qi depression	Treats the six depressions
Xiāo Yáo Sǎn	Liver depression and blood vacuity with vacuity of spleen qi	Headache, irregular menstruation and anorexia
Dān Shēn Yǐn	Cardiac and gastric pain from qi stasis and depressive binding	Costal pain and gastric distress

Discrimination of Prescriptions (*continued*)

Prescription	Pattern	Guiding Symptoms
Yī Guàn Jiān	Insufficiency of liver yin and horizontal counter-flow liver qi	Thoracocostal fullness and pain, acid regurgitation, and bitter taste in the mouth
Lóng Dǎn Xiè Gān Tang	Damp heat in the lower burner and upward counterflow of liver fire	Genital swelling and itching, red eyes, and tinnitus
Dáng Guī Lóng Huì Tāng	Surging of liver fire	Unconsciousness, delirium, and twitching
Xiè Qīng Wán	Liver fire	Vexation, agitation, and fright
Dāng Guī Sì Nì Tāng	Injury by cold to the liver	Cold extremities
Zuǒ Jīn Wǎn	Liver fire	Costal pain, bitter taste in the mouth
Liáng Fù Wán	Liver cold	Stomach pain
Jīn Líng Zǐ Sàn	Depressive stasis from liver qi and liver fire	Costal pain, lateral abdominal distension and pain
Sì Mó Yǐn	Horizontal counterflow of liver qi attacking the stomach, spleen, or lung	Panting [asthma], thoracic fullness
Bái Zhù Sháo Yào Sǎn	Liver effulgence and spleen vacuity	Diarrhea
Wēn Dǎn Tāng	Counterflow of stomach qi and phlegm heat from depression of gallbaldder qi	Vomiting and nausea

5. On the Various Medicinals Commonly Used in Liver Illnesses

Our predecessors categorized the most commonly used medicinal agents in the treatment of liver illnesses. For instance it states in the *Běn Cǎo Gāng Mù*: "The vacuity and repletion of the viscera and bowels provide the parameters for the use of medicinals," and further notes that of the more than seventy kinds of medicinals used in [the treatment of] liver illnesses, all may be divided into the categories of supplementing the blood, supplementing the qi, circulating the qi, calming fright, tracking wind, draining fire and supplementing the mother, and draining the son.

Běn Cǎo Fēn Jīng Shěn Zhì points out that there are many medicinals that enter the liver channel and these may be divided into categories of supplementing, harmonizing, purging, dissipating cold and heat, and so forth.

Nevertheless, in these preceding statements the medicinals for liver illnesses and those that enter the liver channel are not categorized as medicinals with special effects. Moreover, since the nature of these medicinals is complex, they can be applied to the treatment of other viscera and bowels. Yet, we are not saying that there are no medicinals that primarily treat liver illnesses, rather that after mastering [the clinical application of] these medicinal substances, they must be used according to the etiology, pathology, and specific symptoms of any illness.

In studying the medicinal substances used in liver illnesses, and having considered the classifications of our predecessors as a foundation, I have divided them into the six categories of liver supplementing, liver harmonizing, liver coursing, liver clearing, liver warming, and liver calming, which form the foundation for the treatment of liver illnesses. This method of division is presented below.

Supplementing the liver

Medicinals that supplement the liver encompass the categories of nourishing the liver, enriching the liver, and emolliating the liver. Primary among these catgories is nourishment of liver blood. It is not difficult to use methods for supplementing liver blood in all liver vacuity situations. However, care must be taken not to [negatively] influence the movement and transformation functions of the spleen-stomach, nor should this approach become confused with the use of acrid warm and aromatic medicinals used for quickening the blood. Medicinals typically used are as follows:

dāng guī	tangkuei
bái sháo yào	white peony [root]
shú dì huáng	cooked rehmannia [root]
hé shǒu wū	flowery knotweed [root]
shā yuàn zǐ	complanate astragalus seed
gǒu qǐ zǐ	lycium [berry]

And sheep liver (*yáng gān*) and so forth [i.e., other supplementing foods].

Dāng Guī (Tangkuei)

This is the middle section of *dāng guī*. The body is used to supplement blood, the head to arrest bleeding, the tail to circulate the blood, and the entire root to quicken the blood. The body of *dāng guī* is used in blood supplementing prescriptions. It is acrid, aromatic, bitter, and warm, while also being sweet and moistening. It enters the three channels of the heart, liver, and spleen. It is the primary medicinal for supplementing liver blood and is used in all blood vacuity patterns. As the qi and taste tend to be of a warm nature, it is typically used with *bái sháo yào* (white peony [root]), which harmonizes the yin and restrains the yang to regulate and assist its function.

Bái Sháo Yào (White Peony [Root])

There are two kinds of peony, red and white. The white is bitter, neutral, and slightly cold, entering the three channels of the spleen, lung, and liver. White peony is the primary medicinal for nourishing liver yin. It is used extensively in the composition of prescriptions. For supplementing liver blood it is used together with bodies of tangkuei. For coursing liver qi it is used together with *qīng pí* (unripe tangerine peel) and *chái hú* (bupleurum [root]).

In cases of insufficiency of liver blood, the categories of medicinals for emolliating, enriching, and nourishing are essential and must be relied on because the medicinals for coursing the liver and rectifying the qi are mostly acrid, drying, wearing, and dissipating of liver yin. Thus, medicinals from these categories should be used to protect [the liver yin]. *Bái sháo yào* (white peony [root]) is also commonly used in abdominal pain vacuity patterns, because *bái sháo yào* enters the spleen channel and is used to relax the middle. Because liver wood controls the arousal of earth, the liver qi is contracted and the pain resolves of its own accord.

Shú Dì Huáng (Cooked Rehmannia [Root])

Shú dì huáng (cooked rehmannia [root]) is sweet, slightly bitter, and slightly warm. It enters the three channels of the heart, liver, and kidney and is the primary medicinal for supplementing kidney water. Because enriching the kidney nourishes the liver, it is valuable in prescriptions that enrich and supplement liver blood. In general, prescriptions for supplementing the liver first use *hé shǒu wū* (flowery knotweed [root]) and then go further to use *shú dì huáng*. *Běn Cǎo Jiú Zhēn* notes:

> Although shú dì huáng and hé shǒu wū both supplement the yin, they are medicinals for harsh supplementation of the true yin of former heaven and require the combination of medicinals for the supplementation of the constructive blood of latter heaven.

Zhì Hé Shǒu Wū (Processed Flowery Knotweed [Root])

Hé shǒu wū (flowery knotweed [root]) is bitter, astringent, and slightly warm. It enters the two channels of the liver and kidney and is the primary medicinal for the regulation and nourishment of liver blood. In particular, it supplements liver yin and is not cold. It is also able to supplement the yang but is not drying or hot, possessing a moderate and harmonious nature. Nonetheless, it has the side effects of hindering the stomach and lubricating the intestines. It is also contraindicated for use with acrid hot medicinals such as *ròu guì* (cinnamon bark) and *fù zǐ* (aconite [accessory tuber]) unless it is combined with cooked *dì huáng* (rehmannia [root]). Raw, it is very harsh and it lacks the calming, supplementing, and protecting qualities of the prepared medicinal. Fresh, it cools the blood and is a precipitant indicated for wind papules and wind constipation.

Ē Jiāo (Ass Hide Glue)

This is ass hide glue and it is sweet and neutral. Entering the three channels of the lung, liver, and kidney, it enriches and nourishes liver blood, and is simultaneously used to check bleeding. There are a great many kinds of gelatin, all composed of flesh and blood. *Ē jiāo* (ass hide glue) is the most balanced, unlike *lù jiǎo jiāo* (deerhorn glue), which tends to warm the kidney and free the governing vessel, *guī bǎn* (tortoise plastron), which subdues the yang and circulates the conception vessel, *biē jiǎ* (turtle shell), which enriches the yin and clears taxation heat, or *xiá tiān gāo* (beef paste), which supplements the spleen and warms and nourishes the middle qi. Nonetheless, they are [all] difficult to digest due to their sticky and slimy nature and are thus contraindicated in weakness of the spleen and stomach, or are fried with clam powder into beads to diminish their pasty nature. This preparation is called *Ē Jiāo Zhū* (Ass Hide Glue Pellets). For a hemostatic effect it is fried with *pú huáng* (typha pollen).

Shā Yuàn Zǐ (Complanate Astragalus Seed)

This is [also known as] *shā yuàn jí lí* (complanate astragalus seed). Because it is the best medicinal for parturition it is also referred to as *tóng shā yuán* ("child" complanate astragalus)[53] in prescriptions. It is sweet and warm, and supplements the blood, entering the two channels of the kidney and liver. It may be combined with the medicinal for extinguishing wind, *cì jí lí* (tribulus [fruit]), to comprise the combination *Tóng Bái Jí Lì* (Complanate Astragalus and Tribulus Seed).

Gǒu Qǐ Zǐ (Lycium [Berry])

Gǒu qǐ zǐ (lycium [berry]) is sweet and neutral, entering the three channels of the lung, liver, and kidney. It is often used in vacuity of liver and kidney yin and is also capable of slightly assisting the yang qi. Its character is stronger than *shā yuàn zǐ* (complanate astragalus seed) and is an excellent aid to *shú dì huáng* (cooked rehmannia [root]). It is not indicated for use in internal heat conditions. In developing balanced supplementing formulations *gǒu qǐ zǐ* (lycium [berry]) may be combined with *nǚ zhēn zǐ* (ligustrum [fruit]).

Yáng Gān (Sheep Liver)

Sheep liver is bitter and cold, entering the liver channel. It nourishes the liver and clears heat, and is commonly used in liver wind vacuity heat conditions giving rise to ocular redness, heat and pain in the eyes, and blurred vision due to an internal blockage. It is most often administered in pill form or alone as a cooked food.

Medicinals for Supplementing the Liver

Medicinal	Functions	Notes
dāng guī (tangkuei)	Primary medicinal for supplementing liver blood	Warm in nature, used with *bái sháo yào* (white peony [root]) to harmonize the yin and restrain the yang
bái sháo yào (white peony [root])	Primary medicinal for supplementing liver blood	
dì huáng (rehmannia [root])	Primary medicinal for supplementation of kidney water; hence used in prescriptions that supplement liver blood.	
hé shǒu wū (flowery knotweed [root])	Primary medicinal for the regulation and nourishment of liver blood	May injure the stomach; is contraindicated with hot medicinals unless combined with *dì huáng* (rehmannia [root])
ē jiāo (ass hide glue)	Nourishes liver blood and checks bleeding	
shā yuàn zǐ (complanate astragalus seed)	Supplements the blood, enters the liver and kidney channels	
gǒu qǐ zǐ (lycium [berry])	Nourishes liver and kidney yin and assists the yang	Contraindicated in internal heat conditions
yáng gān (sheep liver)	Used in liver vacuity heat patterns manifesting as eye illnesses	

[53]This *"Tóng"* refers to a tributary of the Yellow River. However, without the water radical preceding it, it means a child, a youth.

Liver Harmonization

Liver harmonization encompasses medicinals for quickening the blood such as:

dāng guī	tangkuei
chuān xiōng	ligusticum [root]
chì sháo yào	red peony [root]
bái sháo yào	white peony [root]
dān shēn	salvia [root]
jī xuè téng	millettia [root and stem]
yuè jì huā	China tea rose

It goes further and includes medicinals for circulating the blood and eliminating stasis such as:

hóng huā	carthamus [flower]
táo rén	peach kernel
zé lán	lycopus
chōng wèi zǐ	leonurus fruit
péng é zhú	zedoary

The qi and taste of blood-quickening and blood-circulating medicinals are acrid and warm, and they also have raiding, dissipating, and migratory natures. The pharmacopias refer to these as "blood within qi medicinals." In cases of insufficiency of liver yin and propensity toward stirring of liver yang, calming medicinals must be used. The use of medicinals from the liver harmonizing category is inappropriate because they often cause mental and visual clouding unconsciousness, as well as oral and nasal bleeding. Medicinals for eliminating stasis are rarely used, other than for hard obstructions and menstrual hindrances, and then it is also appropriate to combine them with calming medicinals. In general, blood stasis in liver illnesses implies moving obstructions and inhibitions of blood, as opposed to dissipating an amassment of blood that has become lodged. Therefore, methods that use medicinals that harmonize the blood and quicken the blood are of primary importance.[54]

Dāng Guī (Tangkuei)

In general *dāng guī* (tangkuei) means the entire *dāng guī,* which quickens the blood and regulates menses. It is commonly combined in prescriptions with other medicinals so that, together with *bái sháo yào* (white peony [root]) it harmonizes the blood, and with *chì sháo yào* (red peony [root]), or *chuān xiōng* (ligusticum [root]), it quickens and moves the blood. Other than this, it is combined with *huáng qí* (astragalus [root]), *rén shēn* (ginseng), and *dà huáng* (rhubarb) with the intent of promoting the generation of blood, containing the blood, and eliminating stasis accumulation. Our ancestors referred to *dāng guī* as being able to supplement blood vacuity, moisten blood dessication, free blood stasis, and comfort blood illnesses based on its use in appropriate combinations with other medicinals. From

---

[54]Trans: Blood amassments and tumors require methods specifically for cracking the stasis as opposed to simply quickening the blood. While the medicinals used to crack the stasis, for example, *yù jīn* (curcuma [tuber]), *sān léng* (sparganium [root]), and *hóng huā* (carthamus [flower]) can be found in Qin Bowei's medicinal classes of harmonizing the liver and rectifying the qi, they effectively form a category of their own.

its essential nature, it is said that because it is acrid, disipating, warm, and freeing, it is contraindicated for use in conditions of qi vacuity and exuberance of fire. *Dāng guī wěi* (tangkuei tail) is used to eliminate stasis and *dāng guī xū* (tangkuei fine root) is used to harmonize the network vessels and relieve pain.

Chuān xiōng (ligusticum [root]) has an acrid taste, a warm qi, and is fragrant, entering the liver channel while simultaneously entering the pericardium and gallbladder channels. It ascends to the vertex and descends to the sea of blood, extending laterally to the flesh. This is the most appropiate medicinal whenever there is wind depression and qi stasis resulting in blood obstruction and blood bi. If there are symptoms of blood vacuity, blood dryness, liver fire, or liver yang, this medicinal is contraindicated. Although it is used in *Sì Wù Tāng* (Four Agents Decoction) and *Chuān Xiōng Chá Tiáo Sǎn* (Tea-Blended Ligusticum (Cnidium Root) Powder), it should not be misconstrued as an important medicinal for supplementing the blood or treating headaches.

Chì Sháo Yào (Red Peony [Root])

Bái Sháo Yào (White Peony [Root])

Chì sháo yào (red peony [root]) and *bái sháo yào* (white peony [root]) both enter the blood aspect of the liver channel. *Bái sháo yào* primarily functions to restrain the yin and nourish the constructive, while *chì sháo yào* is used to quicken the blood while simultaneously clearing the blood and dissipating stasis. It is indicated for symptoms of a tendency to effulgence of liver fire. In case of blood vacuity with an effulgence of fire, red peony and white peony may be used together.

Dān Shēn (Salvia [Root])

Dān shēn (salvia [root]) is bitter and slightly cold and enters the two channels of the heart and liver. It quickens the blood, moves the blood, and regulates transportation of the blood fluid. The *Dà Míng* and *Rì Huá* refer to this as "eliminating stasis and engendering the new," with the implication of freeing and supplementing. Salvia is most often used in the treatment of longstanding costal pain and hard obstruction in the early stage.

Jī Xuè Téng (Millettia [Root and Stem])

In harmonizing the blood, *jī xuè téng* (millettia [root and stem]) is best at quickening the network vessels and freeing the channels. Cooked into a paste it is referred to as *Jī Xuè Těng Jiāo* (Millettia Paste) and is particularly strong. Yú Nánzhì refers to this as a great supplementer of qi and blood, being most appropriate in geriatric and gynecological illnesses.

Yuè Jì Huā (China Tea Rose)

Yuè jì huā (China tea rose) is sweet and warm, and capable of soothing the qi and quickening the blood. It is commonly used in gynecology with the intent of freeing the menses.

Hóng Huā (Carthamus [Flower])

Hóng huā (carthamus [flower]) is acrid and warm, entering the liver channel. It is an important medicinal for moving the blood. It is capable of freeing the menses, arresting pain, and dissipating swelling, and is indicated for symptoms relating to stasis and inhibition of the channels and vessels. In general, the most commonly used is *cǎo hóng huā* (carthamus [flower]) which is also refered to as *tǔ hóng huā*. *Xī zàng hóng huā* [the variety of saffron from Tibet] is especially potent. Nonetheless, it moves the blood but does not protect it, and if the intent is to course, free, and harmonize the blood, the dose should not be too large. *Zhū Dānxī* said, "If a lot is used it cracks stasis, and if a small amount is used, it nourishes the blood." This is valuable experience.

Táo Rén (Peach Kernel)

Táo rén (peach kernel) is bitter, neutral, and slightly sweet, entering the two channels of the liver and spleen. It circulates the blood and dispels while simultaneously moistening dryness. Apart from primarily treating hard obstructions and blood amassment, blood [stasis-related] constipation of the large intestine, and menstrual obstruction, it is commonly combined with medicinals for rectifying the qi to effectively treat thoracocostal pain of the network vessels.

Zé Lán (Lycopus)

Zé lán (lycopus) is bitter, acrid, and slightly warm, entering the two channels of the liver and spleen. Moving the blood and eliminating stasis, it is typically used in gynecology for menstrual obstruction. *Běn Cǎo Jīng Sū* says in addition:

> [It] primarily treats enlarged abdomen due to water swelling, superficial edema of the body, face, and extremities, and water qi in the articulations.

Běn Cǎo Jiú Zhēn states: "The flavors enter the spleen and circulate water, enter the liver and treat the blood." Whenever there is depressive stasis of the qi and blood of the liver viscus, which influences the spleen, causing a failure of healthy transportation, and a failure of transformation of water dampness, this medicinal may be considered. It may also be used together with medicinals for the supplementation of the qi and blood, thus supplementing in the midst of dissipation and not causing a wearing depletion of the true source.

Chōng Wèi Zǐ (Leonurus Fruit)

This is the seed of *yì mǔ cǎo* (leonurus). It is a strong blood quickener and circulator like *chōng wèi zǐ* (leonurus fruit), and it is an important medicinal for regulating the menses, which may also be used to downbear water qi.

Péng É Zhú (Zedoary)

Simply called *é zhú* (zedoary), it is bitter, acrid, and warm, entering the liver channel. It cracks stasis and dispells hardness, and is commonly combined with *sān léng* (sparganium [root]) for amassments.

Medicinals for Harmonizing the Liver

Medicinal	Functions	Notes
dāng guī (tangkuei)	Quickens the blood, regulates the menses	Contraindicated for qi vacuity and exuberance of fire
chuān xiōng (ligusticum [root])	Wind depression and qi stasis resulting in blood obstruction	Contraindicated with blood vacuity, blood dryness, liver fire, and liver yang
chì sháo yào (red peony [root])	Quickens the blood and clears blood heat	
jī xuè téng (millettia [root and stem])	Quickens the blood and frees the channels, supplements the qi and blood	Commonly used in gynecology and in geriatrics
yuè jì huā (China tea rose)	Soothes the qi and quickens the blood	Frees the menses in gynecological illnesses
hóng huā (carthamus [flower])	Moves the blood, arrests pain, and dissipates swelling	xī zàng hóng huā (Tibetan saffron) is the most potent
táo rén (peach kernel)	Moves the blood and eliminates stasis while moistening dryness	Treats blood constipation of the large intestine
zé lán (lycopus)	Moves the blood and eliminates stasis and water retention	
chōng wèi zǐ (leonurus fruit)	Strongly quickens the blood and downbears water qi	
é zhú (zedoary)	Cracks stasis and dispells hardness	Combined with sān léng (sparganium [root]) for amassments

Rectification of the Qi

Medicinals for the rectification of qi encompass those for soothing the liver, coursing the liver, and calming the liver, with the intent of regulating the qi and resolving depression. They include the following:

yù jīn	curcuma [tuber]
xiāng yuán	citron
cì jí lí	tribulus [fruit]
chuān liàn zǐ	toosendan [fruit]
jú yè	tangerine leaf
méi guī huā	rose
chái hú	bupleurum [root]
qīng pí	unripe tangerine peel
xiāng fù zǐ	cyperus [root]
yán hú suǒ	corydalis [tuber]
chén xiāng	aquilaria
sān léng	sparganium [root]
mù zéi	equisetum
jú hé	tangerine pip
lì zhī hé	litchee pit

Medicinals for the rectification of the qi are among the most frequently used in the treatment of liver illnesses. Nonetheless, a great many of these [substances] are fragrant, drying, wearing, and dissipating, and are capable of depleting the yin and blood. Thus their use leads to the production of internal heat. The appropriate medicinals must therefore be prescribed based on the severity of the illness, and their use should be discontinued when that is indicated [by the patient's positive response or when side effects appear]. Otherwise, while there may be some immediate positive effect, when injudiciously continued this prescription will only create future suffering.

Yù Jīn (Curcuma [Tuber])

Yù jīn (curcuma [tuber]) is acrid, bitter, and cold, entering the three channels of the heart, liver, and stomach. It is commonly used to treat liver illnesses caused by qi stagnation, with symptoms of thoracocostal fullness, oppression, distension, and pain. Also, beyond being a "qi within the blood medicinal" and rectifying the qi, it is used to dissipate stasis. Therefore, it is most appropriate for depressive binding stasis of qi and blood. In general, *guǎng yù jīn* (southern curcuma [tuber]) is stronger in the elimination of stasis as compared to *chuān yù jīn* (Sichuan curcuma [tuber]).

Xiāng Yuán (Citron)

Xiāng yuán (citron) has an acrid, sour taste, and courses and drains qi stasis in the liver and stomach. It treats distending oppression engendering pain in the thoracocostal and gastric cavities, and is roughly the same as *qīng pí* (unripe tangerine peel) in strength.

Cì Jí Lí (Tribulus [Fruit])

Cì jí lí (tribulus [fruit]) is acrid, bitter, and slightly cold; it courses the liver and drains wind. It is particularly effective in the treatment of all head and eye illnesses, as well as for dispersing wind heat from the liver channel.

Chuān Liàn Zǐ (Toosendan [Fruit])

Chuān liàn zǐ (toosendan [fruit]) is is bitter cold and slightly toxic, capable of coursing depressive binding of fire qi from the liver viscus, as well as draining damp-heat from the bladder. Our ancestors said it either entered the entered the heart and bladder, or that it entered the lung, spleen, and stomach channels, not at all involving the liver channel. Its primary treatment context is as an antiparasitic that treats pain from cardioabdominal shan qi, as well as vague liver illnesses. *Běn Cǎo Fēn Jīng Shěn Zhì* lists it for cold penetration of the liver, and says that it "drains liver fire"; *Zhōng Guó Yī Xué Dá Cí Diǎn* points out that it "enters the four channels of the liver, pericardium, small intestine, and bladder," and the author of that text understands that it "drains liver depression, treats liver qi pain, treats liver qi distension, drains the liver, and drains heat and is an important medicinal for liver channel abdominal pain and shan pain." Based on clinical evidence, *chuān liàn zǐ* (toosendan [fruit]) is used to treat liver qi, internal depression of liver fire precipitating lower abdominal [(i.e., *shào fù*)] distension and pain, shan pain, rough and dark urination, costal pain, and the awareness of pain accompainied by internal heat in the affected area, all to good effect. It is contraindicated in vacuity cold of the intestines and stomach because it can cause loose stools.

Jú Yè (Tangerine Leaf)

Jú yè (tangerine leaf) is bitter and neutral, entering the liver channel while simultaneously entering the stomach channels. It treats costal pain and breast distension and pain in women.

Méi Guī Huā (Rose)

Méi guī huā (rose) is sweet, warm, and slightly bitter, with a fragrant qi entering the two channels of the liver and spleen, soothing the liver and harmonizing the blood, treating liver and stomach qi pain. It is extremely good for regulating and nourishing depressive qi symptoms.

Chái Hú (Bupleurum [Root])

Chái hú (bupleurum [root]) is bitter and slightly cold. Entering the gallbladder channel, it is also used to upbear and dissipate. Used in liver illnesses it primarily courses the qi, resolves depression, and dissipates fire. In prescriptions with medicinals such as *dāng guī* (tangkuei) and *bái sháo yào* (white peony [root]) it rectifies and resolves. *Běn Cǎo Cóng Xīn* mentions that it "diffuses and disinhibits the qi and blood, dissipates binding, and regulates the menses," and states that "everyone knows *chái hú* (bupleurum [root]), promotes the surface, but they often fail to acknowledge that it mostly functions to harmonize the interior."[55] I believe that after all, *chái hú* is a surface medicinal, a medicinal of the qi aspect, and a gallbladder channel medicinal. It is capable of moving the interior, moving the blood aspect, and moving the liver channel, but is entirely dependent upon the medicinals that assist it.

The use of bupleurum by our ancestors was primarily based on specific pathological conditions. They preferred to use it in combination with other medicinals [to achieve the effect they intended], and also had a grasp of the dose appropriate to each [of these] specific uses. Although *chái hú* upbears and dissipates, since the qi and taste are all light, there is no grave risk that it will injure the yin or plunder the fluids. Nevertheless, if there is an insufficiency of liver yin, or ascending counterflow of liver qi, liver fire with symptoms such as headache, tinnitus, dizziness, vomiting, or costal pain, larges doses of *chái hú* may aggravate the intensity of the symptoms, or cause hemorrhage, and therefore caution is advised. Also, *chái hú* is often mentioned in the same breath with other medicinals for coursing the qi such as *qīng pí* (unripe tangerine peel) and *xiāng fù zǐ* (cyperus [root]). They are differentiated in that *chái hú* ascends and dissipates, and is indicated for depressive stasis of the qi mechanism; however, if a horizontal counterflow of liver qi has already occurred, then *qīng pí* and *xiāng fù zǐ* to course and disinhibit are indicated.

Qīng Pí (Unripe Tangerine Peel)

Qīng pí (unripe tangerine peel) is acrid, bitter, and warm, entering the two channels of the liver and gallbaldder. It courses liver qi and is

---

[55]The case is probably the opposite for modern practitioners.

particularly effective in the treatment of costal pain and abdominal distension. If there is concurrent unsoothed stomach qi, then it is combined with *chén pí* (tangerine peel) [the combination of] which is simply called *qīng chén pí*, unripe and ripe tangerine peel.

Xiāng Fù Zǐ (Cyperus [Root])

Xiāng fù zǐ (cyperus [root]) is acrid, slightly sweet, and bitter. It mainly enters the liver channels while simultaneously entering the lung and triple burner channels. It is generally recognized as an important medicinal for rectifying the qi in liver illnesses. Nonetheless, it also rectifies the qi of the triple burner and it is not limited to conditions of liver qi; it harmonizes the blood aspect and is not limited to conditions of the qi aspect. It also has aromatic side effects, and in the presence of vacuity symptoms we should guard against dissipating the qi and wearing the blood.

Yán Hú Suǒ (Corydalis [Tuber])

Yán hú suǒ (corydalis [tuber]) is acrid and warm, simultaneously entering the liver and heart channels. It circulates the blood within the context of qi stasis, and moves the qi within the context of blood stasis. In liver illnesses it is most often used for abdominal pain, typically combined with *chuān liàn zǐ* (toosendan [fruit]).

Chén Xiāng (Aquilaria [Wood])

Chén xiāng (aquilaria [wood]), is acrid and slightly warm, and primarily downbears the qi. *Běn Cǎo Jiú Zhēn* points out:

> Together with *dīng xiāng* (clove) and *ròu guì* (cinnamon bark), *chén xiāng* (aquilaria [wood]) treats eructation from stomach vacuity, and together with *zǐ sū yè* (perilla leaf) and *cǎo dòu kòu* (Katsumada's galangal seed), it treats vomiting due to stomach chill. Together with *fú líng* (poria) and *rén shēn* (ginseng), *chén xiāng* treats insuficieny of heart spirit, and together with *chuān liàn zǐ* (toosendan [fruit]) and *ròu guì* (cinnamon bark) it treats debilitation of life gate fire. Together with *ròu cōng róng* (cistanche [stem]) and *huǒ má rén* (hemp seed), it treats constipation from large intestine vacuity.

In liver illnesses it is most often used to treat worry, depression of the seven affects, qi counterflow, and qi reversal. *Sì Mó Yǐn* (Four Milled Ingredients Beverage) and *Chén Xiāng Huà Zhì Wán* (Aquilaria Stagnation Transforming Pill) with modifications are typical examples of the use of this medicinal. *Jiā nán xiāng*, which is also called *qié nán xiang* (resinous aquilaria [wood]) is an especially potent type of *chén xiāng*. There is also *chén xiāng qū* (aquilaria leaven) which is composed of [the following medicinals]:

chén xiāng	aquilaria [wood]
mù xiāng	saussurea [root]
tǔ huò xiāng	agastache
tán xiāng	sandalwood
jiàng zhēn xiāng	dalbergia [wood]
jiāng huáng	turmeric

xiǎo dòu kòu	Indian cardamom
bái dòu kòu	cardamom
zhǐ ké	bitter orange
qīng pí	unripe tangerine peel
wū yào	lindera [root]
mǔ dān pí	moutan [root bark]
fáng fēng	ledebouriella [root]
qiāng huó	notopterygium [root]
qián hú	peucedanum [root]
gé gēn	pueraria [root]
chái hú	bupleurum [root]
dāng guī	tangkuei
mài yá	barley sprout
gǔ yá	rice sprout
gān cǎo	licorice [root]

This medicinal substance soothes the liver and harmonizes the stomach, courses the surface, and transforms stasis.

Sān Léng (Sparganium [Root])

Sān léng (sparganium [root]) is bitter and neutral. It circulates the qi and arrests pain. Its effect is close to that of *xiāng fù zǐ* (cyperus [root]), but it is more harsh. It is to be used with caution if the body is weak. In the composition of prescriptions it is often combined with *é zhú* (zedoary) in treating masses and accumulations. Because sparganium enters the qi aspect of the liver channel and zedoary enters the blood aspect, they are used to dissipate the qi and crack stasis in both aspects.

Mù Zéi (Equisetum)

Mù zéi (equisetum) is sweet and slightly bitter, entering the two channels of the liver and gallbladder. It courses wind and quickens the blood, upbearing and dissipating depressive fire, and it is an important medicinal in the treatment of reddening of the eyes and distorted vision.

Jú Hé (Tangerine Pip)

Jú hé (tangerine pip) is bitter and neutral, entering the liver channel. It is most often used for shan qi distending pain.

Lì Zhī Hé (Litchee Pit)

Lì zhī hé (litchee pit) is sweet, warm, and astringent, entering the liver. It courses the liver and stomach qi, simultaneously dissipating cold dampness. It is generally used in male shan qi. It is also used to good effect, however, for pain of the abdominal cavity in both men and women. *Lì zhī* (litchee) is sweet and neutral, supplementing the blood and generating liquids. It is also capable of dissipating qi stasis that lacks form[56] and is typically eaten for liver vacuity symptoms in the form of *lóng yǎn ròu* (longan flesh).

---

[56]Qi stasis that lacks form implies a stagnation of qi that has not yet congealed into a physically palpable mass.

Medicinals for Rectifying the Qi

Medicinal	Functions	Notes
yù jīn (curcuma [tuber])	Treats binding stasis of qi and blood	
xiāng yuán (citron)	Courses and drains qi stasis in liver and stomach	
cì jí lí (tribulus [fruit]	Treats wind illnesses in the head	
chuān liàn zǐ (toosendan [fruit])	Antiparasitic, drains liver depression and fire	Contraindicated in vacuity cold of the intestines
jú yè (tangerine leaf)	Treats costal pain and breast distension in women	
méi guī huā (rose)	Soothes the liver and harmonizes the blood in nourishing depressive qi symptoms	
chái hú (bupleurum [root])	Resolves depression, dissipates fire, resolves the surface, and harmonizes interior	Will not injure the yin unless there is a pre-existing insufficiency and symptoms of counterflow
qīng pí (unripe tangerine peel)	Courses the liver in treatment of costal pain	
xiāng fù zǐ (cyperus [root])	Rectifies the qi and harmonizes the blood	Caution as it dissipates the qi and wears the blood in vacuity conditions
yán hú suǒ (corydalis [tuber])	Moves the blood within the qi and the qi within the blood	Specific for treatment of pain
chén xiāng (aquilaria [wood])	Downbears the qi, soothes the liver and harmonizes the stomach	
sān léng (sparganium [root])	Circulates the qi and arrests pain, enters the qi aspect in the treatment of masses and accumulations	Use with caution if the body is weak; sparganium [root] is harsher than cyperus root]
mù zéi (equisetum)	Courses wind and quickens the blood, dissipates depressive fire	Treats red eyes and distorted vision
jú hé (tangerine pip)	Bitter and neutral	Treats shan qi distending pain
lì zhī hé (litchee pit)	Courses the liver and stomach qi while simultaneously dissipates cold	Specific for male shan qi

Clearing the Liver

This category consists of medicinals for clearing the liver. The mild [medicinals] clear liver heat, for example,

mǔ dān pí	moutan [root bark]
huáng qín	scutellaria [root]
shān zhī tàn	charred gardenia [fruit]
xià kū cǎo	prunella [spike]
yīn chén hāo	capillaris
qīng dài	indigo
niú huáng	bovis bile
qīng xiāng zǐ	celosia [seed]
mì méng huā	buddleia [flower]

The strong [medicinals] drain liver fire and are also referred to as "liver-draining medicinals," including substances such as *lóng dǎn* (gentian [root]) and *dàn zhú yè* (bamboo leaf). Medicinals that clear the liver, especially those that drain the liver, are most often bitter cold and injure the stomach. They should be used with caution in cases of weakness of the spleen and stomach.

Mǔ Dān Pí (Moutan [Root Bark])

Mǔ dān pí (moutan [root bark]), is acrid and cold, entering the two channels of the heart and liver. It is the primary medicinal for clearing blood heat from the liver viscus, as well as being an important hemostatic medicinal. Hemostatic medicinals are most often constraining and astringent, but *mǔ dān pí* is capable of simultaneous acrid dissipation without the side effect of congealing and accumulating stasis.

Huáng Qín (Scutellaria [Root])

Huáng qín (scutellaria [root]) is bitter and acrid. It clears heat from the lung, stomach, and large intestine as well as clearing gallbladder fire. The gallbladder is yang and located in the midst of the *jué yīn*, so *huáng qín* (scutellaria [root]) is therefore typically used to treat liver symptoms. It says in *Běn Cǎo Shū Zhēng*:

> For binding heat in the qi aspect, *huáng qín* is coupled with *chái hú* (bupleurum [root]). For binding heat in the blood aspect, *huáng qín* is coupled with *bái sháo yào* (white peony [root]). *Chái hú* is capable of opening the bondage in the qi aspect, but cannot clear the heat of the qi aspect. *Bái sháo yào* is capable of opening the bondage of the blood aspect, but it is unable to clear heat of the blood aspect.

This illustrates the use of *huáng qín* (scutellaria [root]) in the treatment of liver heat illnesses.

Shān Zhī Tàn (Charred Gardenia [Fruit])

Shān zhī tàn (charred gardenia [fruit]) is bitter and cold. It clears fire in the three burners, and treats pathogenic heat with cardiac vexation and agitation. Used in liver illnesses, it is often combined with *huáng qín* (scutellaria [root]) and *qīng hāo yè* (sweet wormwood leaf) to clear the qi aspect, and is combined with *mǔ dān pí* (moutan [root bark]) to clear the blood aspect.

Xià Kū Cǎo (Prunella [Spike])

Xià kū cǎo (prunella [spike]) is bitter, acrid, and cold, entering the channels of both the liver and gallbladder. It clears depressive heat and frees binding qi. Blood dryness or dryness of the liver viscus may produce depressive binding of qi fire, which gives rise to rashes, irrascible temperment, insomnia and many dreams, vexation heat and perspiration, reddening of the eyes, and ocular pain. Because it influences the liver channel, it is efficacious in treating cervical scrofula. Direct cooling and cold methods are not indicated in cases of depressive liver fire. *Xià kū cǎo* (prunella [spike]) is acrid and disipating, but differs from the disipating, upbearing nature of *chái hú* (bupleurum [root]), therefore, it is more appropriate [in these cases].

Qīng Hāo (Sweet Wormwood)

Qīng hāo (sweet wormwood) is bitter and cold with fragrant qi, entering the two channels of the liver and gallbladder. It clears vacuity heat and depressive heat. Many medicinals that are bitter and cold inhibit the spleen and stomach. However, *qīng hāo* is aromatic and pleasing to the spleen, and does not attack the harmony of the middle qi.

Qīng Dài (Indigo)

Qīng dài (indigo) is salty and cold, entering the liver channel. It cools the blood and dissipates heat, while simultaneously resolving toxins. It treats hematemesis due to surging counterflow of liver fire and is generally used in the context of direct bitter cold treatment methods. For longstanding depression of liver heat, with a crimson tongue and red lips, it is generally not sufficient to simply nourish the yin and clear heat, and the use of *dà qīng yè* (isatis leaf) is preferred.

Niú Huáng (Bovis Bile)

Niú huáng (bovis bile) is bitter, neutral, and slightly toxic. It is indicated for use in clearing and resolving when liver heat engenders wind and there is a mutual transformation of wind and fire, causing symptoms of mania-withdrawal and epilepsy. This category of symptoms presents mainly as a combination of heart fire and phlegm heat, and *niú huáng* (bovis bile) simultaneously enters the heart and dissipates phlegm.

Qīng Xiāng Zǐ (Celosia [Seed])

Qīng xiāng zǐ (celosia [seed]) is bitter and slightly cold, entering the liver channel. It is used for reddening of the eyes from wind fire.

Mì Méng Huā (Buddleia [Flower])

Mì méng huā (buddleia [flower]) is sweet, neutral, and slightly cold, entering the liver channel. It is used for reddening of the eyes with copious lacrimation. It is indicated for heat from liver vacuity and indicated in cases of wind fire.

Lóng Dǎn (Gentian [Root])

Lóng dǎn (gentian [root]) is bitter, astringent, and very cold, draining repletion heat from the liver and gallbaldder and clearing damp-heat from the lower burner. In general, when there are symptoms of liver fire, *Lóng Dǎn Xiè Gān Tāng* (Gentian Liver-Draining Decoction) with modifications can be relied upon.

Dàn Zhú Yè (Bamboo Leaf)

Dàn zhú yè (bamboo leaf) is bitter and cold, entering the two channels of the liver and pericardium. It drains the liver and clears heat while simultaneously freeing the stools. It is also used singly to free the stools as in *Gēng Yī Wán* (Toilette Pill).

Medicinals Used in Clearing the Liver

Medicinal	Function	Notes
mǔ dān pí (moutan [root bark])	Clears bood heat from the liver; used for acrid dissipation without the side effect of congelation and stasis	
huáng qín (scutellaria [root])	Clears heat from the lung, stomach, and large intestine and fire from the gallblader	Used in combination with bupleurum for binding heat in the qi aspect and with peony for heat in the blood aspect
shān zhī zǐ (gardenia [fruit])	Clears fire from the three burners	Specific for cardiac vexation and agitation
xià kū cǎo (prunella [spike])	Clears depressive heat and binding qi	To avoid the upbearing nature of *chái hú* (bupleurum) in the treatment of depressive fire, *xià kū cǎo* (prunella [spike]) may be substituted
qīng hāo (sweet wormwood)	Clears vacuity heat and depressive heat, but does not attack the middle qi	
qīng dài (indigo)	Cools blood, clears heat, resolves toxins	Specific for hematemesis from liver fire
niú huáng (bovis bile)	Clears wind caused by liver heat and liver fire	Specific for mania-withdrawal
qīng xiāng zǐ (celosia [seed])	Clears wind fire in the liver channel	Specific for red eyes
mì méng huā (buddleia [flower])	Clears vacuity heat from the liver	Specific for red eyes with lacrimation
lóng dǎn (gentian [root])	Drains repletion heat and damp heat from the lower burner	
dàn zhú yè (bamboo leaf)	Drains the liver and clears heat	Specific for freeing the stools

Warming the Liver

Medicinals for warming the liver include the following:

ròu guì	cinnamon bark
yín yáng huò	epimedium
ài yè	mugwort [leaf]
xiǎo huí xiāng	fennel [fruit]
mù guā	chaenomeles [fruit]

Aside from disipating cold qi from the liver viscus, this category of medicinals also strengthens the liver and is used for insufficiency. Consequently, it supplements the yang of the liver viscus. In prescribing supplementation of liver yang, these warming medicinals must be assisted by those for nourishing the blood because warming medicinals should not be used alone.

Ròu Guì (Cinnamon Bark)

Ròu guì (cinnamon bark) is sweet, acrid, and very warm, entering the three channels of the kidney, liver, and triple burner. *Ròu guì* (cinnamon bark) and *chuān wū tóu* (aconite tuber) are most often referred to as medicinals "for warming the lower burner," because they are used to return the yang and abate the yin. Nonetheless, *chuān wū tóu* supports the original yang and dissipates the yin mist, treating cold reversal. *Ròu guì* frees the blood vessels and dissipates wind cold from the constructive and defensive aspects, treating blood loss due to yin exuberance and menstrual block.

Běn Cǎo Jiú Zhēn points out that *ròu guì* (cinnamon bark) treats blockages in the blood vessels and fortifies the qi and blood. It differs from *chuān wū tóu* (aconite main tuber), which secures the true yang. Therefore, when the qi and blood are disharmonious, and we want them to flow freely, *chuān wū tóu* is not indicated. Moreover, in strongly supplementing the qi and blood, *ròu guì* (cinnamon bark) is added as an assistant such as in *Shí Quán Dà Bǔ Tāng* (Perfect Major Supplementation Decoction) and *Rén Shēn Yǎng Yíng Táng* [also called: *Rén Shēn Yǎng Róng Táng*] (Ginseng Construction-Nourishing Decoction). Because of this, *ròu guì* (cinnamon bark) should be the primary medicinal for warming the liver and dissipating cold, harmonizing the blood, and freeing the vessels. There are a relatively large number of medicinals in the cinnamon family such as *yáo guì* and *méng zì guì* and *yuè nán guì*. The best quality cinnamon is moist, sweet, and aromatic, and is slightly acrid with a dry qi.

Yín Yáng Huò (Epimedium)

Yín yáng huò (epimedium) is acrid, sweet, and warm. It warms and nourishes the liver and kidney, but is not drying. It is most appropriate for all vacuities of the liver viscus.

Ài Yè (Mugwort [Leaf])

Ài yè (mugwort [leaf]) is acrid, bitter, and slightly warm, entering the three channels of the spleen, liver, and kidney. *Ài yè* is used in liver illnesses particularly in gynecology, to warm the uterus and dissipate cold dampness. In general, it is used together with *xiāng fù zǐ* (cyperus [root]), to regulate the menses and arrest abdominal pain, and with *ē jiāo* (ass hide glue) for uterine bleeding during pregnancy and postpartum hemorrhage.

Xiǎo Huí Xiāng (Fennel [Fruit])

There are two kinds of *xiǎo huí xiāng* (fennel [fruit]): large and small, although the type used medicinally is mainly the smaller. It is acrid and dissipates chill qi from the bladder, intestines, and stomach, and in liver illnesses it is used to treat shan qi due to cold congelation qi stasis.

Mù Guā (Chaenomeles [Fruit])

Mù guā (chaenomeles [fruit]) is sour and warm, entering the two channels of the liver and spleen. The liver governs the sinew and this medicinal is used for lack of strength in the lower extremities. It is contraindicated in cases of depressive heat with short, dark urination.

Medicinals for Warming the Liver

Medicinal	Functions	Notes
róu guì (cinnamon bark)	Frees the blood vessels, expels wind cold from the constructive and defensive layers	Used for blood loss and menstrual blockage
fù zǐ (aconite [accessory tuber])	Supports the original yang, dissipates yin mist and treats cold reversal	
yín yáng huò (epimedium)	Warms and nourishes the liver and kidney in all vacuities of the liver viscus	
ài yè (mugwort [leaf])	Warms the uterus and dissipates cold damp	Specific for gynecological liver illnesses
hú lú bā (fenugreek [seed])	Dissipates chill from the bladder and intestines	Specific for shan qi cold stasis
mù guā (chaenomeles [fruit])	Governs the sinew in the treatment of weak lower extremities	Contraindicated in depressive heat patterns with scant dark urine

Calming the Liver

Calming the liver entails subduing the yang [with medicinals] such as:

jú huā	chrysanthemum [flower]
gōu téng	uncaria [stem and thorn]
tiān má	gastrodia [root]
sāng yè	mulberry leaf
mǔ lì	oyster shell
zhēn zhū	pearl Margarita
shí jué míng	abalone shell

This treatment method will further extinguish wind with the additions of *guī bǎn* (tortoise plastron), *biē jiǎ* (turtle shell), *dài mào* (hawksbill [turtle] shell), *líng yáng jiǎo* (antelope horn), *dán cái* (mussel), and so forth.

In cases of liver vacuity with an upward harassment of wind yang and a tendency to heat, medicinals are used that have a cooling nature, and [that] are also referred to as "medicinals for cooling the liver." At the same time because of the arousal of a blood yin insufficiency or internal heat resulting in yin vacuity, these are typically combined with medicinals for supplementing the blood and enriching the yin. Aside from these, we have medicinals for tracking wind that are, in general, also referred to as "medicinals for extinguishing wind." Two examples are *gān xié* (scorpion) and *wú gōng* (centipede), and these are used differently.[57]

Jú Huā (Chrysanthemum [Flower])

Jú huā (chrysanthemum [flower]) is bitter and neutral, entering the channels of the heart, liver, spleen, lung, stomach, and large intestine. In terms of liver illnesses it is of primary importance for clearing the head and eyes in [treating] symptoms such as headaches, head distension, cephalic dizziness, visual dizziness, and reddening of the eyes. There are many kinds of *jú huā* (chrysanthemum [flower]). The flower from Háng Zhōu, which is small and yellow in color, is the main one, while the white flowers are relatively sweet and warm. The flowers from Chú Zhōu are also white and taste bitter at first, then sweet, and have an especially clearing, aromatic qi. Therefore, there are the following:

háng jú	Hangzhou chrysanthemum [flower]
huáng jú huā	yellow chrysanthemum [flower]
bái jú huā gēn	white chrysanthemum root
jú huā	chrysanthemum [flower]
jú huā	Chuzhou chrysanthemum [flower]

They are named as such when composing prescriptions.

Gōu Téng (Uncaria [Stem and Thorn])

Gōu téng (uncaria [stem and thorn]) is sweet and slightly cold, entering the two channels of the heart and liver. It clears fire and settles wind, and treats liver heat dizziness and fright convulsions. Its qi is mild and if the illness is severe, then *gōu téng* cannot address it.

Tiān Má (Gastrodia [Root])

Tiān má (gastrodia [root]) is acrid and neutral, entering the liver channel. It settles an internal stirring of wind and is indicated for dizziness from blood vacuity. Our predecessors refered to it as coursing wind, transforming phlegm, and diffusing and freeing the channels and network vessels [when used] in the treatment of wind strike paralysis. They also asserted that it treats internal wind rather than external wind.

Sāng Yè (Mulberry Leaf)

Sāng yè (mulberry leaf) is bitter, sweet, and cold, entering the three channels of the lung, stomach, and large intestine. It courses wind and clears heat. While it is basically a medicinal for symptoms of superficial external afflictions, it is also capable of clearing depressive heat in the liver and gallbladder, brightening the eyes, and eliminating distending pain in the head and brain.

---

[57]While medicinals for extinguishing wind and tracking wind are often the same, Qin Bowei has not taken pains to discriminate between the two treatment principles (see "Tracking the Liver," p. 40). Scorpion and centipede are in the class of medicinals for calming the liver in general; however they are specifically indicated for tracking wind.

Mǔ Lì (Oyster Shell)

Mǔ lì (oyster shell) is salty, neutral, and slightly cold, entering the three channels of the kidney, liver, and triple burner. Raw, it is used to subdue the yang; calcined, it is used to secure and astringe. Raw *mǔ lì* is [the form] most commonly used in liver illnesses for the treatment of liver yang cephalic dizziness. Since salty flavors are able to soften hardness, it is used for scrofula. For subcostal pi lumps it must be accompanied by *chái hú* (bupleurum [root]) as a guide. Oyster flesh, known as *lì huáng,* is sweet and warm and is enriching and supplementing. It is best used as an assistant for agitation of liver yang from blood vacuity.

Guī Bǎn (Tortoise Plastron)

Guī bǎn (tortoise plastron) is sweet, neutral, salty, and cold. It nourishes the yin and subdues the yang, and is used for symptoms of liver wind. The gelatin known as *guī bǎn jiāo* (tortoise plastron glue) is especially potent.

Biē Jiǎ (Turtle Shell)

*Biē jiǎ (*turtle shell), is salty and neutral, entering the liver and simultaneously entering the channels of the spleen and lung. It enriches the yin and subdues the yang, abating bone steaming, and also treating masses and accumulations and malarial lump glomus. *Biē jiǎ* (turtle shell) is commonly used together with *mǔ lì* (oyster shell) and *guī bǎn* (tortoise plastron). In *Wēn Bìng Tiáo Biàn,* *Sān Jiǎ Fù Mài Tāng* (Triple-Armored Pulse-Restorative Decoction) is used for warm pathogens transforming and entering the lower burner, injuring the yin and blood of the liver and kidney. First, *mǔ lì* (raw oyster shell) is used, next *biē jiǎ* (raw turtle shell), and finally *shēng guī bǎn* (raw tortoise plastron) is used. This illustrates the use of sequencing [specific medicinals over the course of treatment]. Use of *guī bǎn* (tortoise plastron) and stewed *biē jiǎ jiāo* (turtle shell glue) is especially potent for enriching and supplementing.

Dài Mào (Hawksbill [Turtle] Shell)

Dài mào (hawksbill [turtle] shell) is sweet and cold. When employing medicinals for clearing heat and resolving toxins, our ancestors believed that this could be employed in the same manner as *xī jiǎo* (rhinoceros horn). Nonetheless, its use clinically is very effective in treating blood vacuity cephalic dizziness, clarifying its use for subduing yang and extinguishing wind.[58]

Líng Yáng Jiǎo (Antelope Horn)

Líng yáng jiǎo (antelope horn) is salty and cold, entering the liver channel and simultaneously entering the lung and heart channels. It is a potent medicinal for extinguishing wind, clearing heat, and calming the liver. It says in *Běn Cǎo Gāng Mù:*

---

[58]Trans: The ancients used *dài mào* (hawskbill [turtle] shell) much like *xī jiǎo* (rhinoceros horn). *Dài mào* also addresses patterns of blood vacuity that *xī jiǎo* does not. This makes *dài mào* particularly useful in pattens involving wind in ascendent yang, which by definition exhibit an element of vacuity.

*The liver governs wood, opens the orifice of the eyes, and in ill-
nesses of the eye such as visual dimness and cataract, líng yáng
jiǎo (antelope horn) calms the liver. The liver governs wind and
meets the sinew, so when illness develops such as infantile fright
epilepsy, pregnancy epilepsy, major wind strike convulsive spasm
resulting in sinew contracture, and all kinds of contracture pain,
líng yáng jiǎo (antelope horn) soothes it. The hún [ethereal soul]
is the spirit of the liver and when illness develops such as fright
and agitation, manic excesses, and eccentricities, líng yáng jiǎo
calms them. The blood is stored by the liver and when illness
develops, such as stasis pouring downward, shan pain, toxic
dysentery, swellings and sores, scrofula, and postpartum blood
and qi stagnation, líng yáng jiǎo dissipates it. The ministerial
fire lies in the liver and gallbladder and creates anger in the qi
level. When illness develops producing vexation and fullness with
qi counterflow, hiccuping obstruction, chills and fever resulting
from injury by cold, and deep-lying fever, then líng yáng jiǎo
downbears it.*

In summarizing its effects, it is primarily clearing and calming.

Zhēn Zhū (Pearl Margarita)

Zhēn zhū (pearl) is sweet, salty, and cold. It clears liver fire in the
treatment of cephalic dizziness, tinnitus, and also spirit-disposition symptom patterns from an effulgence of heart and liver fire. Although it enters
the liver channel, it is not the same as *shí jué míng* (abalone shell).

Shí Jué Míng (Abalone Shell)

Shí jué míng (abalone shell) is salty and neutral, entering the liver
channel. It is most effective for visual dizziness and reddening of the eyes
from liver heat generating wind. Since the nature of its effects are close
to those of *mǔ lì* (oyster shell) and *zhēn zhū* (pearl), the three are often
used together when composing prescriptions [that pertain to the pattern of
liver heat generating wind]. Nonetheless, one should guard against [the]
needless duplication [of these medicinals].

Dán Cái (Mussel)

Mussel is sweet and warm. It treats emaciation and dizziness from liver
vacuity, and is capable of enriching the yin and subduing the yang. Yè
Tiānshì used it to treat symptoms of liver wind, and also referred to it as *dán
cái jiǎo* (mussel gelatin). *Rì Huá Běn Cǎo* states, "eating too much of this
medicinal will cause a person to have oppression and blurring of the head
and eyes." However, this has no basis in clinical practice.

Quán Xiē (Scorpion)

Quán xiē (scorpion) is sweet, acrid, neutral, and toxic. It enters the liver
and tracks wind in the treatment of straying vision, shaking of the head,
and contracture of the hands and feet. In general, it is said that [tracking
wind is fundamentally] different from extinguishing wind. In the composition of prescriptions, *quán xiē* (scorpion) [and *xiē wěi* (scorpion tail)] are
most often used because all the substance's potency is in the tails.

Wú Gōng (Centipede)

Wú gōng (centipede) is acrid, warm, and toxic. It tracks pathogenic
wind from the liver viscus, and its effects are close to those of *quán xiē*
(scorpion).

Medicinals for Calming the Liver

Medicinal	Function	Notes
jú huā (chrysanthemum [flower])	Clears the head and eyes	Specific for headache, dizziness, and red eyes
gōu téng (uncaria [stem and thorn])	Clears fire and settles wind, treats liver heat dizziness	This is a relatively mild medicinal
sāng yè (mulberry leaf)	Courses wind, clears heat, clears vacuity heat, and brightens the eyes	Specific for distending pain in the head and brain
mǔ lì (oyster shell)	Raw, it subdues the yang; calcined, it secures and astringes	
guī bǎn (tortoise plastron)	Nourishes the yin and subdues the yang in the treatment of liver wind symptoms	
biē jiǎ (turtle shell)	Enriches the yin and subdues the yang	Specific for bone steaming and masses and accumulations
dài mào (hawksbill [turtle] shell)	Subdues the yang and extinguishes wind in the treatment of mental dizziness due to blood vacuity	Is a substitute for xī jiǎo (rhinoceros horn)
líng yáng jiǎo (antelope horn)	Extinguishes wind, clears heat, and calms the liver	Treats fright epilepsy, wind strike, and contracture pain
zhēn zhū (pearl Margarita)	Drains an effulgence of liver and heart fire	Treats mental dizziness, tinnitus, and spirit disposition symptoms
shí jué míng (abalone shell)	Drains liver heat generating wind	Visual dizziness and red eyes
dán cái (mussel)	Enriches the yin and subdues the yang	Treats emaciation, dizziness, and blurring vision
quán xiē (scorpion)	Tracks wind	Treats straying vision, contracture, and spasms
wú gōng (centipede)	Tracks wind	Treats straying vision, contracture, and spasms

The above enumeration of sixty-four ingredients does not embrace all the medicinals commonly used in liver illnesses. There are a great many medicinals that do not enter the liver channels but that are nonetheless used in treating liver illnesses and these have not been mentioned here. In studying medicinal substances we must understand their basic functions, how they are used in combination, and what it is they primarily treat, as well as their auxilliary uses.

For instance, in the case of chái hú (bupleurum [root]), it is important to understand the functions of its flavor as a single ingredient. It is also important to understand its use in combination with bái sháo yào (white peony [root]) and huáng qín (scutellaria [root]). It is important to understand its strong points, and it is important to understand that its ascending and dissipating qualities can cause injury. If the quality and use of *chái hú* (bupleurum [root]), is neglected [in composing prescriptions], and its medicinal utility is judged solely based on its use in *Xiǎo Chái Hú Tāng* (Minor Bupleurum Decoction) and *Xiāo Yáo Sǎn* (Free Wanderer Powder) this is an obvious mistake. If *chái hú* is thought of only in terms of its ability to course the liver and we [thus] fail to consider that the manner in which it is typically used often plunders the yin, this is also unsatisfactory. This principle should not be applied only to medicinals for liver illnesses but for all medicinals as well.

Summary

I may have rambled in completing this talk. Particularly in my failure to advance a single treatment method and prescription for any single illness, I may not have satisfied everyone's needs. My main intent in explaining the treatment of liver illnesses has not been to delineate commonly used prescriptions. For that matter, we cannot cling to [the idea of using only] prescriptions specifically designed for liver illnesses [in treating liver illnesses]. We must go beyond theory to the discrimination of patterns, and from there to the excecution of prescription methods in actual therapy.

Is this discussion aiming too high in laying particular emphasis on theory? It is not! If there is a comprehensive understanding of the treatment of liver illnesses, as well as a comprehensive grasp of the methodology applied, then the essential theory of liver illnesses will be integrated into treatment. The facts tell us that if a person in clinical practice thinks only in terms of prescriptions for liver illnesses, this is not only inflexible and limiting, but prevents progress in considering simple illnesses by making them more difficult and thus makes understanding complex illnesses impossible. For example, if only *Xiāo Yáo Sǎn* (Free Wanderer Powder) is employed in the treatment of costal pain, and if it is used entirely and not modified according to the circumstances, success cannot be achieved and one will be left helpless without a viable strategy. As an example of the combination of theory and clinical experience, Yè Tiānshì's treatment of costal pain used prescription methods of acrid warm [medicinals for] freeing the network vessels, sweet relaxing [medicinals for] rectifying vacuity, warm emolliating [medicinals to] free and supplement, and acrid and draining [medicinals] to diffuse stasis. [Yè Tiānshì's] use of medicinals to compose prescriptions was naturally also meticulous and skillfull.

In terms of recent therapies for the treatment of liver illnesses in modern times, Yè Tiānshì was very skillfull and moreover [from his thoughts about] a simple pattern a single emcompassing law of therapy emerges. Huá Xuíyún detailed and summarized liver wind, liver fire, and liver depression, and wood overwhelming earth. This may be referred to in *Lín Zhèng Zhǐ Nán Yī Àn* for [further] study. Naturally, it is also important to read medical books to promote progressively deeper and broader treatment of liver illnesses.

(March 1962)

An Informal Discussion on the Use of Medicinals in Prescription

Because they are so familiar, I do not intend to discuss the [famous] general methods such as the seven prescriptions and ten formulas.[1] In today's discussion I would like to examine a few of the issues involved in the practical application [of Chinese medicine], embracing the principle of "saying all you know and saying it without reserve," by offering a critique of this approach. It is expected that you, my students, will assume the attitude of "correcting mistakes, if any exist, and guarding against making any [of your own,] if there are none."

1. Application of Medicinals in Prescriptions is Rationally Based

The application of medicinals in prescription is rationally based, that is, treatment proceeds [logically] from a discrimination of patterns. In a rationally based approach to the administration of prescriptions and medicinals, it is of essential importance that one "state the rationale, establish the treatment methods, select a prescription, and consider the use of specific medicinals." In terms of treatment based on pattern identification, pattern identification seeks to determine a cause. Having examined the disease factor, one then discusses treatment. Selection of a prescription [then proceeds] on the basis of the methods chosen; then the discussion of specific medicinals to be used [that follows] is based on the prescription selected. Using this approach, it is obvious whether or not the medicinals in a prescription and the symptoms are in accord, whether or not the medicinals have been carefully combined, whether or not the doses are appropriate, and whether or not there is a sequential pattern to the arrangement of the medicinal substances [used]. All these aspects are used to evaluate the level of understanding applied in the composition of a prescription.

---

[1]*Chinese-English–English-Chinese Terminology of Chinese Medicine,* published by Hunan Science and Technology Press, defines the seven prescriptions only as an ancient Chinese classification comprised of seven classes. The Ten Formulas or prescriptions classified dissipators, mobilizers, supplements, purgatives, light and heavy prescription lubricants, astringents, dessicants, and moisteners.

The intent of a prescription is to treat an illness and, therefore, the medicinals used must derive from [an evaluation of] the disease factor, location of the disorder, and symptoms of the root illness. As a result, the organization of a prescription encompasses the three aspects that can be conveyed in a formula:[2]

DISEASE FACTOR + LOCATION OF THE DISORDER + SYMPTOMS [= PATTERN = FORMULA]

The disease factor is the original source of the disorder, while the location of the disorder is where the illness lies. These two [factors] should be clearly understood because they are the focus of our thinking in using medicinals. The symptoms are the overall presentation of the pathogenic condition and, with treatment, the symptoms will most often disappear once the disease factor disappears. Although treatment is derived from pattern identification, [which is] based on the symptoms [expressed in an illness] in clinical practice, we are not usually limited to considering only symptoms when composing a prescription. Nevertheless, where symptoms do exist and, furthermore, when the patient is in pain and suffering from spiritual distress, then appropriate consideration must be given [to these symptoms and treatment should be] based on the intensity of those symptoms, as they increase, decrease, or change entirely.

In discussing treatment methods, the *Nèi Jìng* notes, "If it is cold, heat it, if it is hot, cool it," which pertains to the disease factor. It also states, "If it is elevated, then dissipate it; if it is low, guide and exhaust it; if there is fullness in the middle, drain the interior." This pertains to the location of the illness. It further states, "If it is dispersed, then contract it; if it is disturbed, then balance it; if there is urgency, relax it." This pertains to the symptoms.

The essential connection to make here is that the treatment of symptoms must not deviate from the [treatment of the] disease factor and the location of the disorder or "patholocale." The disease factor and the location of the illness are the root and the symptoms are the branch. In the final analysis, this is nothing other than "the necessity of seeking the root in treating illness."

Take, for example, a patient with aversion to cold, scratchy throat, copious thin white phlegm, a floating slippery pulse, and a slimy white tongue coat. The diagnosis is wind-cold cough with loss of the functions of diffusion and transformation of lung qi. In using medicinals in prescription it is essential that all the aspects – coursing wind and dispersing cold, diffusing the lung, and transforming phlegm to suppress cough – be addressed by the prescription. Those aspects may be assimilated in our example formula in the following way:

COURSE AND DISPERSE WIND COLD + DIFFUSE THE LUNG + TRANSFORM PHLEGM TO SUPPRESS COUGH [= COMPREHENSIVE TREATMENT METHODS]

The use of medicinals in prescription must not deviate from these therapeutic protocols and parameters. For instance, *Xīng Sū Sǎn* (Apricot Kernel and Perilla Powder) is typically employed [in cases such as those

---

[2]Trans: Qin is using an algebraic model to reflect the rational power inherent in each step of the T.C.M. method. In the original text he leaves the outcome of each equation implied but unstated, as teachers sometimes do to stimulate their student. Thus, hoping to make reading easier, we have inserted the outcomes in square brackets.

described above] and it is organized as follows: The prescription contains *zǐ sū yè* (perilla leaf) and *qián hú* (peucedanum [root]), which are acrid and wind-cold dispersing, entering the lung channel, while *qián hú* simultaneously downbears the qi and transforms phlegm. *Xìng rén* (apricot kernel), *jié gěng* (platycodon [root]), *zhǐ ké* (bitter orange), and *gān cǎo* (licorice [root]) are used in combination to diffuse the lung and regulate the qi of the chest. *Bàn xià* (pinellia [tuber]), *chén pí* (tangerine peel), and *fú líng* (poria) are used to transform phlegm, normalize the qi, and suppress cough. This can also be described in the following manner:

zǐ sū yè   (perilla leaf)
qián hú   (peucedanum [root])

+

xìng rén (apricot kernel)
jié gěng (platycodon [root])
chén pí (tangerine peel)
gān cǎo (licorice [root])

+

bàn xià (pinellia [tuber])
qīng pí (unripe tangerine peel)
fú líng (poria)

[=]

[*Xīng Sū Sǎn* (Apricot Kernel and Perilla Powder)]

In this example, we can understand the major methods of prescription composition and the major questions involved. First, prescription composition is based on clearly defined treatment methods. Thus, it has a fixed focus and scope and the use of medicinals necessarily reflects the three aspects of the illness – disease factor, location, and symptom pattern – [which indicates that] the medicinals should all work together in concert. For instance, *qián hú* (peucedanum [root]) disperses wind-cold but is also able to downbear the qi and transform phlegm. *Xìng rén* (apricot kernel) perfuses the lung but is also able to normalize the qi and suppress cough.

[Second,] having analyzed the organization of the medicinal substances in the standard prescriptions cited [in the prescription literature], appropriate modifications based on the presenting symptoms can be made to produce an even more intimate [relation to the patient's condition]. For instance, in the absence of thoracic fullness and oppression, *zhǐ ké* (bitter orange) may be deleted and, in the absence of copious turbid phlegm, *bàn xià* (pinellia [tuber]) and *fú líng* (poria) may also be deleted. In addition, the lung-perfusing, phlegm-transforming properties of *niú bàng zǐ* (arctium [seed]) and *bèi mǔ* (fritillaria [bulb]), and the throat-moistening, cough-suppressing properties of *pàng dà hài* (sterculia) may all be incorporated into the prescription.

Third, based on the principle noted above, any formulation may be used that is in accord with treatment methods for addressing the root illness. If the formulation is not in accord with these treatment methods, this is obvious at a glance. For instance, if one does not use *Xīng Sū Sǎn* (Apricot Kernel and Perilla Powder) it is appropriate to use *Sān Ào Tāng*

(Rough and Ready Three Deoction) for, although the ingredients are quite simple, *má huáng* (ephedra) enters the lung and disperses cold, while *xìng rén* (apricot kernel) perfuses the lung, normalizes the qi, and suppresses cough.[3] Both [medicinals] address the disease factor and location of the illness, while also giving therapeutic consideration to the symptoms. This is what makes *Sān Ào Tāng* an efficacious prescription for cough from external contraction. On the other hand, *Yín Qiào Sǎn* (Lonicera and Forsythia Powder) is used for external contraction of wind-warm and, although it perfuses and transforms the upper burner, it is not in accord with the salient disease factor [in this example], and it is naturally inappropriate.

Fourth, consideration of the symptoms must be based on a consideration of the fundamental [problem]. [Simply because] the root and branch are integrated, does not necessarily imply a symptomatic treatment. For instance, the focus in cough from external contraction is coursing the pathogen. For that reason, medicinals for calming cough are not used. Rather, if the exogenous pathogen is resolved, and the lung qi cleared and perfused, then the phlegm and cough disappear on their own and the effect of the treatment will be surprisingly good.

These principles are all based on the guiding theories of Chinese medicine. The use of medicinals in composing prescriptions must be based on these principles and the arguments here presented are thus also based on them.

2. A GRASP OF THE FUNDAMENTAL TREATMENT METHODS IS HELPFUL IN USING MEDICINALS IN PRESCRIPTIONS

To ensure the mature composition of prescriptions in clinical practice, we must firmly grasp the fundamental treatment methods, encompassing [an understanding of] general therapeutic methods such as those regarding disease factor and symptom pattern. Although [discussions of] these therapeutic methods are present throughout the literature, an effort must nonetheless be made to collate these materials, and to skillfully prepare strategies that are adaptable to the changing conditions [of a patient's illness]. For instance, when vacuity patterns are encountered, it is generally understood that supplementation is indicated. It is understood that in spleen vacuity the spleen is supplemented, and that in kidney vacuity the kidney is supplemented. Furthermore, we understand sayings such as:

> . . . *in supplementing of the spleen why not supplement the kidney, and in supplementing of the kidney why not supplement the spleen?*

> . . . *an effulgence of earth generates metal, so do not be restricted to protecting metal; an effulgence of water extinguishes fire, so do not avidly clear the heart.*

> . . . *in nourishing the spleen, the lung must not be hindered; in enriching the kidney, the spleen must not be impeded.*

---

[3]Trans: *gān cǎo* (licorice [root]) is present in this prescription as an envoy to harmonize the influence of the other medicinals and to moderate the diaphoretic effect of the *má huáng* (ephedra). The entire formula is taken as a draught with five slices of *shēng jiāng* (fresh ginger). Clearly, Qin Bowei considers these ingredients as merely adjunctive to the ephedra.

Nevertheless, in actual therapeutic experience, because symptom presentations tend to be complex, we often become confused or decide that there is a paucity of [relevant] treatment methods and [thus that] no established prescription is appropriate. It is my belief that the nature of a vacuity must be determined to properly apply a supplementing formula. [We must ask] in what viscera is the vacuity? To what degree is there vacuity? Furthermore, the direction from which the supplementation originates must be considered. Should direct prescription methods be used, while simultaneously using indirect methods? If supplementation is used, will there or will there not be harmful reactions?

If we want to settle this series of questions, we must first understand the cause of the vacuity. What variety of symptoms are present in this vacuity pattern? What mechanism is at work in the vacuity pattern within the affected internal viscera and what is it influencing in turn? [By answering these questions] we can establish the nature of the standard supplementation formula to be used, as well as the compatibilities and contraindications of the medicinal substances of which it is composed.

Now, I will illustrate my experience in using medicinals in the composition of prescriptions for enriching and nourishing the qi and yin in the treatment of vacuity patterns. Methods for enriching and nourishing the qi and yin are of primary importance in cases of insufficiency of lung qi and lung yin. These insufficiencies are predominantly due to a lingering of warm pathogens, flaring of fire from the five dispositions, wearing dispersion of the qi aspect and burning consumption of the fluids. Because there is a vacuity of both qi and yin [that is] creating a failure of the function of pulmonary depuration, consequent symptoms such as shortness of breath, dry cough with scant sticky phlegm, hacking blood, and dry mouth are often seen.[4] In addition to these symptoms, because the lung rules the skin and hair, an insecurity of defensive qi will also manifest through symptoms of copious perspiration and aversion to wind.

In the case of lung supplementation, in addition to discriminating between medicinal substances that supplement the qi and those that supplement the yin, it is also important that we be familiar with those medicinal substances that are used for suppressing cough, transforming phlegm, and checking sweating in lung vacuity patterns. Moreover, because the lung has relationships with the heart, liver, spleen, and kidney, we are also likely to see symptoms such as cardiac vexation, palpitations, insomnia, irascibility, tidal fevers, and loose stool. These relationships need to be expanded to include consideration of those medicinal substances that address the other related internal organs and [those] that are also specifically appropriate for lung vacuity.

Enriching and nourishing the qi and yin is a major therapeutic method and, when using medicinals in a prescription, this series of questions [noted above] must be considered. In this way, if we grasp the fundamental

---

[4]Trans: Symptom pattern syllogisms are inherently vague in Chinese. The relationship of cause and effect, pattern and symptom, derives from the epistemology of the more organic Chinese view of the universe. Thus, definition of a cause and effect relationship is to some extent interpretation, not translation, and the English must be left somewhat open. This is particularly true in the classical language. In this case, stating that the failure of pulmonary depuration causes the symptoms does no harm to the expression's clinical validity.

treatment methods and adopt the fundamental formulas and medicinal substances, then we are possessed of a complete understanding and [will] use medicinals in prescription in a mature way. Also, as to enriching and nourishing the qi and yin, a few medicinals are explained in the chart that follows:

Action	Medicinal
Supplement Lung Qi	huáng qí (astragalus [root])
	rén shēn (ginseng)
	xī yáng shēn (American ginseng)
Supplement Lung Yin	běi shā shēn (glehnia [root])
	mài mén dōng (ophiopogon [tuber])
	tiān huā fěn (trichosanthes root)
	bǎi hé (lily bulb)
Suppress Cough	xìng rén (apricot kernel)
	pí pá yè (loquat leaf)
	mǎ dōu líng (aristolochia fruit)
	hē zǐ (chebule)
Transform Phlegm	bèi mǔ (fritillaria [bulb])
	hǎi gé ké (clamshell)
	dōng guā zǐ (wax gourd seed)
	yì yǐ rén (coix [seed])
Hemostatic	xiān hè cǎo (agrimony)
	cè bǎi yè (biota leaf)
	qiàn cǎo gēn (madder [root])
	ǒu jié (lotus root node)
	mǔ dān pí (moutan [root bark])
Allay Thirst	lú gēn (phragmites [root])
	bái máo gēn (imperata [root])
Check Sweating	fú xiǎo mài (light wheat [grain])
	sāng yè (mulberry leaf)
	wǔ wèi zǐ (schisandra [berry])
Clear the Liver	qīng dài (indigo)
	huáng qín (scutellaria [root])
	xià kū cǎo (prunella [spike])
Enrich the Kidney	shēng dì huáng (rehmannia [root])
	biē jiǎ (turtle shell)
	tiān mén dōng (asparagus [tuber])
Support the Spleen	shān yào (dioscorea [root])
	bái zhú (ovate atractylodes [root])
	biǎn dòu (lablab [bean])
	gān cǎo (licorice [root])

As for prescriptions, Zhāng Jǐngyuè's *Xīn Fāng Bā Zhèn (Eightfold Array of New Prescriptions)* and *Gǔ Fāng Bā Zhèn (Eightfold Array of Ancient Prescriptions)* are in the supplementing array *[bǔ zhèn].* But beyond formulas in the category of lung supplementation, it is also important to be familiar with the harmonization array *[hé zhèn]* and the cold array *[hán zhèn]*, which are [also] related to lung vacuity formulas. For example:

***Sì Yīn Jiān* (Four Yin Decoction) contains:** *shēng dì huáng* (dried/fresh rehmannia [root]), *mài mén dōng* (ophiopogon [tuber]), *běi shā shēn* (glehnia [root]), *bái sháo yào* (white peony [root]), *bǎi hé* (lily bulb), *fú líng* (poria), and *gān cǎo* (licorice [root]).

***Mài Mén Dōng Yín Zī* (Ophiopogon Drink) contains:** *mài mén dōng* (ophiopogon [tuber]), *huáng qí* (astragalus [root]), *rén shēn* (ginseng), *dāng guī* (tangkuei), *shēng dì huáng* (dried/fresh rehmannia [root]), and *wǔ wèi zǐ* (schisandra [berry]).

***Ē Jiāo Sǎn* (Ass Hide Glue Powder) contains:** *ē jiāo* (ass hide glue), *bái jí* (bletilla [tuber]), *tiān mén dong* (asparagus [tuber]), *wǔ wèi zǐ* (chisandra [berry]), *rén shēn* (ginseng), *shēng dì huáng* (dried/fresh rehmannia [root]), and *fú líng* (poria).

***Tiān Mén Dōng Wán* (Asparagus Pills) contains:** *tiān bèi mǔ* (fritillaria [bulb]), *xìng rén* (apricot kernel) , *ē jiāo* (ass hide glue), *fú líng* (poria), and *gān cǎo* (licorice [root]).

***Lù Yún Sǎn* (Green Cloud Powder) contains:** *cè bǎi yè* (biota leaf), *rén shēn* (ginseng), *ē jiāo* (ass hide glue), and *bǎi hé* (lily bulb).

***Rén Shēn Qīng Fèi Tāng* (Ginseng Lung-Cleansing Decoction) contains:** *rén shēn* (ginseng), *xìng rén* (apricot kernel), *ē jiāo* (ass hide glue), *yīng sù qiào* (poppy [husk]), *gān cǎo* (licorice [root]), *sāng bái pí* (mulberry root bark), *zhī mǔ* (anemarrhena [root]), *dì gǔ pí* (lycium root bark), and *wū méi* (mume [fruit]).

***Rén Shēn Píng Fèi Sǎn* (Ginseng Lung-Calming Decoction) contains:** *rén shēn* (ginseng), *tiān mén dōng* (asparagus [tuber]), *huáng qín* (scutellaria [root]), *dì gǔ pí* (lycium root bark), *chén pí* (tangerine peel), *qīng pí* (unripe tangerine peel), *fú líng* (poria), *zhī mǔ* (anemarrhena [root]), *wǔ wèi zǐ* (schisandra [berry]), *gān cǎo* (licorice [root]), and *dì gǔ pí* (lycium root bark).

***Èr Mǔ Sǎn* (Anemarrhena and Fritillaria Powder) contains:** *bèi mǔ* (fritillaria [bulb]) and *zhī mǔ* (anemarrhena [root]).

***Zǐ Wǎn Sǎn* (Aster Powder) contains:** *zǐ wǎn* (aster [root]), *ē jiāo* (ass hide glue), *zhī mǔ* (anemarrhena [root], *bèi mǔ* (fritillaria [bulb]), *rén shēn* (ginseng), *gān cǎo* (licorice [root]), *fú líng* (poria), *jié gěng* (platycodon [root]), and *wǔ wèi zǐ* (schisandra [berry]).

***Yù Quán Wán* (Jade Spring Pill) contains:** *rén shēn* (ginseng), *mài mén dōng* (ophiopogon [tuber]), *huáng qí* (astragalus [root]), *fú líng* (poria), *wū méi* (mume [fruit]), *gān cǎo* (licorice [root]), *tiān huā fěn* (trichosanthes root), and *gé gēn* (pueraria [root]).

Even with an understanding of fundamental formulas and medicinal substances, there are still many aspects of our ancestral experience to absorb, such as an understanding of what is indicated and what is to be avoided [in the use of medicinals]. For instance, *Dān Xī Xīn Fǎ* points out:

> *With a dry mouth and throat and phlegm, do not use bàn xià (pinellia [tuber]) or tiān nán xīng (arisaema [root]). Use guā lóu (trichosanthes [fruit]) and bèi mǔ (fritillaria [bulb]) instead.*

Also,

> *Xìng rén (apricot kernel) drains the lung qi, so in the case of long-standing cough from qi vacuity, discontinue its use after one or two administrations.*

Also,

> *Yīng sù qiào (poppy [husk]) is frequently used in the treatment of cough. It is important, however, to eliminate the root illness first, and it is to be used only after other medicinals [have been tried.]*

And,

> *Zhī mǔ (anemarrhena [root]) suppresses cough and clears the lung, moistens yin, and downbears fire.*

In sum, it is important to understand the standard methodology and it is also important to understand more subtle modifications, not only to minimize error in using medicinals in prescriptions but also so that these methods can be explained once a therapeutic effect has been obtained.

3. THE SKILLFUL USE OF ESTABLISHED PRESCRIPTIONS

Established prescriptions *[chéng fāng]* are the prescriptions of our ancestors that have been handed down to us by virtue of their effectiveness in practice. Thus, they deserve additional attention because they are important for learning the proper use of medicinals in prescriptions. To be competent in prescription composition we must memorize many prescriptions, [they are] like capital [upon which to draw].[5] Nevertheless, [among such] established prescriptions there are prescriptions for general treatment *[tōng zhì fāng]* and prescriptions which govern treatment *[zhǔ zhì fāng]*. These must be clearly distinguished.

What does "general treatment" or "governing or primary treatment" mean? Xú Língtāi states:[6]

> *A single illness must have a single prescription, and the specific treatment used is referred to as the "governing prescription [zhǔ fāng]." Furthermore, a single illness also has several subcategories and each subcategory also has a governing prescription.*

He also states,

> *. . . a governing prescription is a specific treatment for a single illness, while a prescription which treats a great variety of illnesses is referred to as a prescription for general treatment.*

---

[5]Trans: The character here is in fact the "capital" of capitalist economics. Although this does seem an odd use in a Communist milieu, socialist thinkers also need a concept for accumulated value that can be drawn down or applied.

[6]Trans: This is the pen name of Xu Dachun, the famous classical writer mentioned in the Introduction as one of Qin's predecessors in the development of medical literature. The quotation here is from the text translated as, Unschuld P.U., *Forgotten Traditions of Ancient Chinese Medicine,* Brookline, Massachusetts: Paradigm Publications, 1990.

As a result of this [traditional distinction, the text] *Lān Tái Guǐ Fàn* is divided into general treatments and those related to specific diseases. It is my feeling that general prescriptions and specific prescriptions should each have their own distinct characteristics and, while prescriptions for general treatment may also be associated with specific representative illnesses, they nevertheless possess a broader therapeutic scope. If these prescriptions for general use are used with proper modifications, then this [too] provides an appropriate foundation for using medicinals in prescription. If, on the contrary, they are used indiscriminately and are only superficially understood, they simply become vulgarized.

For instance, *Liù Wèi Dì Huáng Wán* (Six Ingredient Rhemannia Pill) principally treats a depletion of kidney yin that gives rise to symptoms of emaciation and lumbar pain. The [prescription] literature states that it treats liver and kidney insufficiency and is supposed to treat the three yin as well. In addition to spontaneous perspiration and thief perspiration, it treats water flood [*shuǐ fàn,* edema] causing phlegm, seminal emission, hemafecia, sore throat, and toothache. It treats all these things but, when all is said and done, we must recognize the primary disease factor, the primary viscera affected, and the primary symptoms [and then] modify the formula based on our experience treating the pathological condition [manifest by the patient]. For instance, if someone believes that yin vacuity patterns can all be treated generally, and [therefore] they invariably use *Liù Wèi Dì Huáng Wán* for these patterns, the therapeutic effect will definitely not be good.

Our ancestors treated taxation cough due to a joint vacuity of lung and kidney yin with the additions of *mài mén dōng* (ophiopogon [tuber]) and *wǔ wèi zǐ* (schisandra [berry]), which is known as *[Bā Xiān] Cháng Shòu Wán* (Eight Immortals Longevity Pill). Visual dizziness and clouding confusion due to dual liver and kidney yin vacuity were treated with the additions of *gǒu qǐ zǐ* (lycium [berry]) and *jú huā* (chrysanthemum [flower]), which is known as *Qí Jú Dì Huáng Wán* (Lycium Berry, Chrysanthemum, and Rehmannia Pill). Soreness and pain of the low back and knees from constitutional weakness was treated through the addition of *dù zhòng* (eucommia [bark]) and *tǔ niú xī* (native achyranthes [root]). Urinary frequency was treated by the additions of *cǎo dòu kòu* (Katsumada's galangal seed) and, as well, the deletion of *zé xiè* (alisma [tuber]). Therefore, I believe that the use of medicinals in prescription should depend on established prescriptions; however, each specific use must be independently considered. In this we can unceasingly strive to create new applications based on the foundations laid by the skill of our ancestors.

It is common knowledge that *Zuǒ Guī Yǐn* (Left-Restoring [Kidney Yin] Beverage) and *Zuǒ Guī Wán* (Left-Restoring [Kidney Yin] Pill) are both famous formulas for supplementation and are stronger than *Liù Wèi Dì Huáng Wān* (Six Ingredient Rhemania Pill). *Zuǒ Guī Yǐn* is in fact *Liù Wèi Dì Huáng Wán* with the deletion of *mǔ dān pí* (moutan [root bark]) and *zé xiè* (alisma [tuber]), and the addition of *gǒu qǐ zǐ* (lycium [berry]) and *gān cǎo* (baked licorice [root]). *Zuǒ Guī Wán* is *Liù Wèi Dì Huáng Wán* with the deletions of *mǔ dān pí* (moutan [root bark]), *zé xiè* (alisma [tuber]), and *fú líng* (poria), and the addition of *gǒu qǐ zǐ* (lycium [berry]), *lù jiǎo jiāo* (deerhorn glue), *guī bǎn* (tortoise plastron), *tù sī zǐ* (cuscuta [seed]), and *tǔ niú xī* (native achyranthes [root]).

Zhāng Jǐngyuè has stated, " . . . use the implications of the six tastes but do not use the six taste prescription itself." Although the primary ingredients of *Liù Wèi Dì Huáng Wán* (Six Ingredient Rhemanina Pill) are basically unchangeable, it is quite natural to strive for new heights [in clinical practice] by sifting through the old [books] to discover new para-meters for current use. At the same time, [Jǐngyuè] specifically described how these prescription methods are to be used in the clinic. When *Zuǒ Guī Wán* (Left-Restoring [Kidney Yin] Pill) is used in the presence of lung heat and vexation, *mài mén dōng* (ophiopogon [tuber]) is added. *Bǎi hé* (lily bulb) is added in cases of lung heat and copious cough. *Bái sháo yào* (white peony [root]) is added in the case of splenic heat and hunger; *xuán shēn* (scrophularia [root]) is added in the case of cardiac heat and severe agita-tion. *Dì gǔ pí* (lycium root bark) is added in cases of renal heat and bone steaming. *Nǚ zhēn zǐ* (ligustrum [fruit]) is added in the case of unsettled yin vacuity and *dì huáng* (raw rehmannia [root]) is added for cases of fre-netic blood heat. When *Zuǒ Guī Wán* is used in cases of dry stools, *tù sī zǐ* (cuscuta [seed]) is deleted and *ròu cōng róng* (cistanche [stem]) is added. *Gǒu qǐ zǐ* (lycium [berry]) and *lù jiǎo jiāo* (deerhorn glue) are deleted and *nǚ zhēn zǐ* (ligustrum [fruit]), and *mài mén dōng* (ophiopogon [tuber]) are added for cases of upflaming of vacuity fire. It can be seen [from these examples that] these prescriptions are quite flexible when used clinically for specific cases.

Based on the inspiration of Zhāng Jǐngyuè, I propose that when we use an established prescription, we must analyze the primary treatment [method implicit in the formula] and primary medicinals used. At the same time, the prescription must be modified based on the patient's spe-cific pathological condition. For instance, *Guī Sháo Dì Huáng Tāng* (Tangkuei, Peony, and Rehmannia Decoction) treats symptoms of liver and kidney yin vacuity, and is *Liù Wèi Dì Huáng Wán* (Six Ingredient Rehmannia Pill) with the additions of *dāng guī* (tangkuei) and *bái sháo yào* (white peony [root]). While *dāng guī* (tangkuei) and *bái sháo yào* (white peony [root]) are naturally the primary medicinals for supplement-ing liver blood, the primary medicinals for supplementing kidney yin are *dì huáng* (prepared rehmannia [root]) and *shān zhū yuí* (cornus [fruit]). These four substances can be regarded as the fundamental medicinals of the prescription. Furthermore, consider the similarities in the use of *gǒu qǐ zǐ* (lycium [berry]), *nǚ zhēn zǐ* (ligustrum [fruit]), *hé shǒu wū* (flowery knotweed [root]), and *ē jiāo* (ass hide glue) in assisting the enrichment and supplementation of kidney yin and blood. The primary therapeutics of the source prescription do not change and it remains amply potent. Another aspect of this prescription is that it places heavy emphasis on enrichment and supplementation of the liver and kidney [and thus] balances the var-ious aspects of its supplementation while emphasizing the general supple-menting measures. This must be decided by considering the pathological condition. Three separate formulae can be used to understand the combi-nation of medicinals in this prescription.

1. Joint methods for supplementing the liver and kidney

The prescription of general treatment lays equal stress on the liver and kidney. *Shān zhū yú* (cornus [fruit]), *gǒu qǐ zǐ* (lycium [berry]), and *nǚ zhēn zǐ* (ligustrum [fruit]) [enrich the kidney yin] and *dāng guī* (tangkuei), *bái sháo yào* (white peony [root]), *hé shǒu wū* (flowery knotweed [root]), and *ē jiāo* (ass hide glue) [enrich the liver blood].

2. Methods for enriching the kidney and emolliating the liver

In the prescription for general treatment [it is] enriching the kidney [that] is primary, assisted by nourishing the liver. *Shú dì huáng* (cooked rehmannia [root]), *shān zhū yú* (cornus [fruit]), *gǒu qǐ zǐ* (lycium [berry]), and *nǚ zhēn zǐ* (ligustrum [fruit]) [to enrich the kidney], plus *dāng guī* (tangkuei) and *bái sháo yào* (white peony [root]) [to nourish the liver].

3. Methods for supplementing the mother when there is vacuity of the son

In the prescription for general treatment [it is] supplementing the liver [that] is primary, while the kidney is simultaneously enriched. *Dāng guī* (tangkuei), *bái sháo yào* (white peony [root]), *hé shǒu wū* (flowery knotweed [root]), and *ē jiāo* (ass hide glue) [emphasize liver supplementing, while] *dì huáng* (prepared rehmannia [root]) and *shān zhū yú* (cornus [fruit]) [enrich the kidney].

Medicinals for enriching the liver and kidney are not limited to these categories, nor are their combinations limited to these mechanisms. Furthermore, in determining what effects we might expect of a given formula, we must look at the strength of the medicinal substances themselves and the dose that will be used [in actually administering the formula to the patient]. An assessment cannot be made solely on the quality of the medicinal flavors.

These examples are used only for illustration. The foundations of established prescriptions rest upon appropriate modification and [thus] an appropriate discrimination of the primary and secondary issues must be simultaneously considered. Nevertheless, although there are variations on this source prescription, it is basically a prescription for general treatment. Because vacuity of liver and kidney yin can produce a variety of disease patterns, the specific disease pattern that the prescription actually treats cannot be sufficiently clear [from the formula alone]. In cases of cephalic dizziness, visual dizziness, and tinnitus, *guī bǎn* (tortoise plastron), *mǔ lì* (oyster shell), *jú huā* (chrysanthemum [flower]), and *tiān má* (gastrodia [root]) are added [to the base prescription *Liù Wèi Dì Huáng Wán* (Six Ingredient Rehmannia Pill)]. In the case of afternoon tidal fever, burning heat in the palms, and copious perspiration, medicinals such as *biē jiǎ* (turtle shell), *mǔ dān pí* (moutan [root bark]), *dì gǔ pí* (lycium root bark), and *bái wéi* (baiwei [cynanchum root]) are added [to the base prescription *Liù Wèi Dì Huáng Wán*].

Because therapy is intimately connected to the presenting symptoms, a prescription for general treatment may be transformed into a prescription governing (specific) treatment. This use of medicinals in prescription is routine but it is only when we understand the ins-and-outs of these routine skills of [prescription] modification that we can encompass the entire condition and move beyond outer appearances. Naturally, once an appropriate established prescription has been chosen and modified, we must attend to the auxiliary actions of the medicinal substances and to the patient's constitution. For instance, the nature of *shú dì huáng* (cooked rehmannia [root]) is warm, enriching, and greasy. *Shēng dì huáng* (fresh rehmannia [root]) is indicated for a patient with internal heat. In cases where a weakness of the stomach and intestines has been observed, *shēng dì huáng tàn* (charred dried rehmannia [root]) may be used or *bái dòu kòu* (cardamom) may be admixed. The old doctors have abundant experience of this variety and their work must be studied carefully.

Beyond this, selection of an established prescription most often proceeds from recognition of the primary pattern. Although this has been discussed above, the disease factor and the location of the illness also occupy important positions in the process of composing a prescription. We must attend to whether or not the disease factor and location of the illness are in accord [with the pattern for which the established prescription is appropriate]. For instance, if the primary patterns are similar and the disease factor, or the location of the illness, does not match [what is expected], a prescription based on that pattern cannot be used. On the other hand, if the disease factor and the location of the illness are in accord, but the salient symptoms do not cohesively match [the disease factor and the location of the illness], then this is a situation that certainly merits close consideration. [For example,] I have used *Huáng Qí Jiàn Zhōng Tāng* (Astragalus Center-Fortifying Decoction) in the treatment of gastric pain from vacuity cold and I have also used *Guì Zhī Tāng* (Cinnamon Twig Decoction), with the addition of *huáng qí* (astragalus [root]) and *dāng guī* (tangkuei) to treat patients with a weakened constitution and a propensity to contracting colds that cause arthritic soreness and pain. I have obtained good results in this way. Expanding upon this, I typically use a formula for disorders on the exterior of the body *[wài kē], Yáng Hé Tāng* (Harmonious Yang Decoction), in the treatment of stubborn phlegm rheum, cough, and asthma, the effect of which is superior to that of *Xiǎo Qīng Lóng Tāng* (Minor Green-Blue Dragon Decoction).

The grounds [for this application] are quite simple. *Xiǎo Qīng Lóng Tāng* treats phlegm rheum cough and asthma due to wind-cold. The disease factor and pathology of *Yáng Hé Tāng* (Harmonious Yang Decoction) and that of phlegm rheum are virtually identical and, moreover, it integrates the capacity to address the copious phlegm. We see in these [examples] an ample illustration of what is called the "agile utilization of established prescriptions," not only with respect to modifications, but also, and most importantly, in the context of the theories guiding independent evaluation and the ability to employ [these established prescriptions] with wide-ranging versatility.[7] As a result of this, we must acknowledge that if we attach importance to primary symptoms but ignore the disease factor

---

[7]Trans: Qin's point here is that we need not be constrained by a limited number of established formulas for any given pattern. A clear understanding of the etiology, location, and patterns involved in a given disease, combined with an intimate familiarity with the organization of a wide range of prescriptions, allows us to select the most appropriate prescription for any given illness regardless of the indications of the prescription chosen.

and the location of the disorder, we are attending to trifles and neglecting the essentials. We must also understand that not only are prescriptions used in this way but medicinals are also used in the same way. Lately there are those who speak of medicinal substances only in terms of what they mainly treat. They fail to give any attention to their qi, taste, or entering channel. Although I believe that it is important to discuss the primary [conditions that a medicinal] treats, the qi, taste, and entering channel cannot be ignored lest the discrimination of patterns determining treatment become disjointed.

4. ATTENDING TO THE COMBINATION OF MEDICINAL SUBSTANCES

Dāng guī (tangkuei) and *bái sháo yào* (white peony [root]) are frequently used together in prescription, as are *cāng zhú* (atractylodes [root]) and *hòu pò* (magnolia bark), or *bàn xià* (pinellia [tuber]) and *qīng pí* (unripe tangerine peel). When combining medicinal substances in this way, the accumulated experience of our ancestors is of principal importance, because it is based in theory, and is not simply a random assemblage [of empirical tricks].

The effectiveness of medicinal substances can be enhanced by appropriate combinations, thus extending the scope of therapy, and this deserves our attention. So that everyone may grasp this, and to promote further understanding of their use, I have drafted descriptions of three categories [of medicinal combination], which are listed below.

Category One

This category consists of combinations of two medicinals that have a dissimilar nature, [for example,] dissimilar qi and taste. Substances are combined with other substances that exhibit dissimilar functions, such as those affecting qi with those affecting blood, those that are cold with those that are hot, those that supplement and [those that] drain, those that disperse with those that contract [*shōu*], those that upbear with those that downbear, and those that are acrid with those that are bitter, and so forth. Combining medicinal substances that are opposed but complimentary changes the original effect and creates new results. This category is the most significant.

Opposed But Complimentary Medicinal Substances in Combination

Type	Example	Function
Guì Zhī (Cinnamon Twig) with *Bái Sháo Yào* (White Peony [Root])		
qi-blood	*Guì Zhī Tāng* (Cinnamon Twig Decoction)	Regulation and harmonization of constructive and defensive
Rén Shēn (Ginseng) with *Dān Shēn* (Salvia [Root])		
qi-blood	*Èr Shēn Dān* (Two Spirits Pill)	Nourishes the heart, harmonizes the blood
Chuān Liàn Zǐ (Toosendan [Fruit]) with *Yán Hú Suǒ* (Corydalis [Tuber])		
qi-blood	*Jīn Líng Zǐ Sǎn* (Toosendan Powder)	Relieves abdominal pain

Xiāng Fù Zǐ (Cyperus [Root]) with *Gāo Liáng Jiāng* (Lesser Galangal Root)

qi-blood	*Liáng Fù Wán* (Lesser Galangal and Cyperus Pill)	relieves gastric pain

Shān Zhī Zǐ (Gardenia [Fruit]) with *Mǔ Dān Pí* (Moutan [Root Bark])

qi and blood	*Jiā Wèi Xiāo Yáo Sǎn* (Supplemented Free Wanderer Powder)	Clears liver heat

Huáng Lián (Coptis [Root]) with *Ròu Guì* (Cinnamon Bark)

cold-hot	*Jiāo Tai Wán* (Peaceful Interaction Pill)	Treats insomnia from lack of communication between the heart and kidney

Huáng Lián (Coptis [Root]) with *Wú Zhū Yú* (Evodia [Fruit])

cold-hot	*Zuǒ Jīn Wán* (Left-Running Metal Pill)	Calms liver and controls eructation

Huáng Lián (Coptis [Root]) with *Gān Jiāng* (Dried Ginger)

cold-hot	*Xiè XīnTāng* (Heart Draining Decoction)	Rids pathogenic binding from the chest

Shì Dì (Persimmon Calyx) with *Dīng Xiāng* (Clove)

cold-hot	*Dīng Xiāng Shì Dì Tāng* (Clove and Persimmon Decoction)	Arrests counterflow belching

Shí Gāo (Gypsum) with *Xì Xīn* (Asarum)

cold-hot	*Èr Xīn Sǎn* (Two Acrid Ingredient Powder)	Eliminates gingival swelling and pain

Huáng Lián (Coptis [Root]) with *Mù Xiāng* (Saussurea [Root])

cold-hot	*Xiāng Lián Wán* (Saussurea and Coptis Pill)	Arrests red and white dysentery

Huáng Lián (Coptis [Root]) with *Hòu Pò* (Magnolia Bark)

cold-drying	*Lián Pǒ Sǎn* (Coptis and Magnolia Bark Powder)	Transforms dampness and heat in the spleen and stomach

Huáng Bǎi (Phellodendron [Bark]) with *Cāng Zhú* (Atractylodes [Root])

cold-drying	*Èr Miào Wán* (Mysterious Two Powder)	Treats damp heat in the lower burner

Bái Zhú (Ovate Atractylodes [Root]) with *Zhǐ Ké* (Bitter Orange)

supplementing-dispersing	*Zhī Zhù Wán* (Unripe Bitter Orange and Ovate Atractylodes Pill)	Strengthens the spleen and disperses pi

Huáng Qí (Astragalus [Root]) with *Fáng Fēng* (Ledebouriella [Root])

supplementing-dispersing	*Yù Píng Fēng Sǎn* (Jade Wind-Barrier Powder)	Treats common cold with bodily vacuity

Bái Sháo Yào (White Peony [Root]) with *Chái Hú* (Bupleurum [Root])

supplementing-dispersing	*Sì Nì Sǎn* (Counterflow Cold Powder)	Harmonizes the liver and discharges heat

Dà Zǎo (Jujube) with *Shēng Jiāng* (Fresh Ginger)

supplementing-dispersing	*Guì Zhī Tāng* (Cinnamon Twig Decoction)	Harmonizes the qi and blood

Biē Jiǎ (Turtle Shell) with Qīng Hāo Yè (Sweet Wormwood Leaf)		
supplementing-clearing	Qīng Hāo Bēi Jiǎ Tāng (Sweet Wormwood and Turtle Shell Decoction)	Abates bone steaming

Zhī Má (Sesame [Seed]) with Sāng Yè (Mulberry Leaf)		
supplementing-clearing	Sāng Má Wán (Mulberry Leaf and Sesame Pill)	Treats liver yang cephalic dizziness

Gǒu Qǐ Zǐ (Lycium [Berry]) with Jú Huā (Chrysanthemum [Flower])		
supplementing-clearing	Qí Jú Dì Huáng Wán (Lycium Berry, Chrysanthemum, and Rehmannia Pill)	Brightens the eyes

Gān Jiāng (Dried Ginger) with Gǒu Qǐ Zǐ (Lycium [Berry])		
dissipating-contracting	Líng Gān Wǔ Wèi Jiāng Xīn Tāng (Poria [Hoelen], Licorice, Schisandra, Ginger, and Asarum Decoction)	Transforms phlegm rheum

Bái Fán (Alum) with Yù Jīn (Curcuma [Tuber])		
constraining-dissipating	Bái Jīn Wán (Alum and Curcuma Pill)	Treats epilepsy

Chái Hú (Bupleurum [Root]) with Qián Hú (Peucedanum [Root]		
upbearing-downbearing	Bài Dú Sǎn (Toxin-Vanquishing Powder)	Courses pathogen and suppresses cough

Jié Gěng (Platycodon [Root]) with Zhǐ Ké (Bitter Orange)		
upbearing-downbearing	Xīng Sū Sǎn (Apricot Kernel and Perilla Powder)	Regulates qi obstruction of the chest and diaphragm

Bàn Xià (Pinellia [Tuber]) with Huáng Qín (Scutellaria [Root])		
acrid-bitter	Xiè Xīn Tāng (Heart-Draining Decoction)	Arrests vomiting

Zào Jiǎo Cì (Gleditsia Thorn) with Bái Fán (Alum)		
acrid-sour	Xī Yán Sǎn (Drool-Thinning Powder)	For frothy vomit from wind phlegm

Wū Méi (Mume [Fruit]) with Xiān Dì Huáng (Fresh Rehmannia [Root])		
sour-sweet	Lián Méi Tāng (Coptis and Mume Decoction)	Transforms the yin and generates fluids

Wū Méi (Mume [Fruit]) with Huáng Lián (Coptis [Root])		
sour-bitter	Lián Méi Tāng (Coptis and Mume Decoction)	Discharges vexation heat

Dāng Guī (Tangkuei) with Bái Sháo Yào (White Peony [Root])		
moving-calming	Sì Wù Tāng (Four Agents Decoction)	Nourishes and harmonizes the blood

Category Two

This category consists of combinations of two medicinal substances that assist one another and are circulating. Their respective strong points are given free reign, and are enhanced when used together, such as combining medicinals for transforming dampness and rectifying the qi; or combining those [medicinals] that promote diaphoresis and free the yang;

those that encompass upbearing and downbearing properties; those that combine exterior and interior effects; or those that combine for mutual intensification and potentization. Combinations in this category are the [ones] most often used clinically, for instance:

Medicinal Combination	Formula Example Function
cāng zhú (atractylodes [root]) and *hòu pò* (magnolia bark)	*Píng Wèi Săn* (Stomach-Calming Powder)
	Dries dampness and circulates the qi
dòu chǐ (fermented soybean) and *xiè bái* (Chinese chive [bulb])	*Cōng Chǐ Tāng* (Scallion and Fermented Soybean Decoction)
	Dissipates cold and frees the yang
bàn xià (pinellia [tuber]) and *chén pí* (tangerine peel)	*Èr Chén Tāng* (Two Matured Ingredients Decoction)
	Transforms phlegm and normalizes the qi
xìng rén (apricot kernel) and *bèi mǔ* (fritillaria [bulb]	*Sāng Xìng Tāng* (Mulberry Leaf and Apricot Kernel Decoction)
	Normalizes qi and transforms phlegm
zhī mǔ (anemarrhena [root]) and *bèi mǔ* (fritillaria [bulb])	*Èr Mǔ Săn* (Anemarrhena and Fritillaria Powder)
	Clears heat and transforms phlegm
zhǐ shí (unripe bitter orange) and *zhú rú* (bamboo shavings)	*Wēn Dǎn Tāng* (Gallbladder-Warming Decoction)
	Harmonizes the stomach and arrests vomiting
mù xiāng (saussurea [root]) and *bīn láng* (areca [nut])	*Mù Xiāng Bīng Láng Wăn* (Saussurea and Areca Pills)
	Circulates the qi and frees stagnation
rén shēn (ginseng) and *gé jiè* (gecko)	*Rén Shēn Gē Jiè Săn* (Ginseng and Gecko Powder)
	Absorbs the qi
huáng qí (astragalus [root]) and *fáng jǐ* (fangji)	*Huáng Qí Fáng Jǐ Tāng* (Astralagus and Fangji Decoction)
	Circulates epidermal edema
rén shēn (ginseng) and *fù zǐ* (aconite [accessory tuber])	*Shēn Fù Tàng* (Ginseng and Aconite Decoction)
	Warms and supplements the original qi
huáng qí (astragalus [root]) and *fù zǐ* (aconite [accessory tuber])	*Qí Fù Tāng* (Astragalus and Aconite Decoction)
	Warms and secures the defensive qi
cāng zhú (atractylodes [root]) and *fù zǐ* (aconite [accessory tuber])	*Zhù Fù Tāng* (Ovate Atractylodes and Aconite Decoction)
	Warms and supplements the middle qi
fù zǐ (aconite [accessory tuber]) and *fú líng* (poria)	
	Potentiation; warms the kidney, disinhibits water
huáng bǎi (phellodendron [bark]) and *zhī mǔ* (anemarrhena [root])	
	Mutual intensification; clears dampness and heat from the lower burner

Category Three

[This category] includes combinations of medicinal substances that have similar natures and effects, and that are used together with the intent of enhancing the effect of [each of] the medicinals, or giving simultaneous consideration to effects on two internal organs. For instance:

Combination	*Explanation*
dǎng shēn (codonopsis [root]) *huáng qí* (astragalus [root])	Supplements the qi
fù zǐ (aconite [accessory tuber]) *ròu guì* (cinnamon bark)	Warms the kidney and returns the yang
shān yào (dioscorea [root]) *biǎn dòu* (lablab [bean])	Supplements the spleen and arrests diarrhea
běi shā shēn (glehnia [root] *mài mén dōng* (ophiopogon [tuber])	Moistens the lung and generates fluids
bǎi zǐ rén (biota seed) *suān zǎo rén* (spiny jujube [kernel])	Nourishes the heart and calms the spirit
dù zhòng (eucommia [bark] *xù duàn* (dipsacus [root])	Supplements the kidney and strengthens the lumbar
huǒ má rén (hemp seed) *guā lóu zǐ* (trichosanthes seed) (typically rendered in prescription as *luó má rén)*	Moistens the intestines and promotes the stools
lóng gǔ (dragon bone) *mǔ lì* (oyster shell) (typically rendered in prescription as *duàn lóng mǔ)*	Secures desertion
jīn yīng zǐ (Cherokee rose fruit) *qiàn shí* (euryale [seed]	Secures the essence
chì shí zhī (halloysite) *yǔ yú liáng* (limonite)	Astringes the intestines
gǔ yá (rice sprout) *mài yá* (barley sprout) (typically rendered in prescription as *gǔ mài yá)*	Assists digestion
sāng zhī (mulberry twig) *sī guā luò* (loofah)	Quickens the network vessels
mǔ lì (oyster shell) *shí jué míng* (abalone shell)	Restrains the yang
shēng má (cimicifuga [root]) *chái hú* (bupleurum [root])	Upbears the qi aspect
xuán fù huā (inula flower) *dài zhě shí* (hematite)	Downbears the qi
jú hé (tangerine pip) *lì zhī hé* (litchee pit)	Disperses shan qi
gān sōng (nardostachys [root]) *shān nài* (kaempferia [root])	Relieves gastric pain
hǎi zǎo (sargassum) *hǎi kūn bù* (kelp)	Disperses phlegm nodules
sān léng (sparganium [root]) *é zhú* (zedoary)	Disperses concretions and accumulations and pi lumps
bái fú líng (white poria) *chì fú líng* (red poria) (typically rendered in prescription as *chì bái líng)*	Disinhibits water

gān suì zǐ (Kansui radix) *yuán huā* (genkwa [flower])	Expels water
cháng shān (dichroa [root]) *bái dòu kòu* (cardamom)	Terminates malaria
dāng guī (tangkuei) *chuān xiōng* (ligusticum [root])	Quickens the blood and rids stasis
táo rén (peach kernel) *hóng huā* (carthamus [flower])	Cracks stasis
rǔ xiāng (frankincense) *mò yào* (myrrh) (typically rendered in prescription as *zhì rǔ mò*)	Rectifies the qi, dissipates stasis, and relieves pain
huò xiāng (agastache) *pèi lán* (eupatorium) (typically rendered in prescription as *huà pèi lán)*	Clears summerheat
jīn yín huā (lonicera [flower]) *lián qiáo* (forsythia [fruit])	Clears heat and resolves toxins
huáng lián (coptis [root]) *huáng qín* (scutellaria [root])	Drains fire
sāng yè (mulberry leaf) *qiāng huó* (notopterygium [root]) *dú huó* (tuhuo [angelica root]) (typically rendered in prescription as *qiāng dú huó)*	Treats wind damp soreness and pain
chuān wū tóu (aconite main tuber) *fù zǐ* (aconite accessory tuber) (typically rendered in prescription as *chuān cǎo wū*)	Treats cold damp soreness and pain
qīng pí (unripe tangerine peel) *chén pí* (tangerine peel) (typically rendered in prescription *qīng chén pí*)	Courses the liver and rectifies the qi
zǐ sū gěng (perilla) *huò xiāng gěng* (agastache/patchouli) (typically rendered in prescription as *sū huò gěn*)	Rectifies the spleen and stomach qi
tiān mén dōng (asparagus [tuber]) *mài mén dōng* (ophiopogon [tuber]) (typically rendered in prescription as *tiān mài dōng)*	Enriches and nourishes the lung and kidney
lú gēn (phragmites [root]) *máo gēn* (imperata [root]) (typically rendered in prescription as *lú mǎo gēn)*	Clears lung and stomach heat
bái dòu kòu (cardamom) *shā rén* (amomum [fruit]) (typically rendered in prescription as *shā kòu rén*)	Strengthens the spleen and stomach
shén qū (medicated leaven) *shān zhā* (crataegus [fruit])	Disperses digestate accumulations of grains and meat

While the above examples of medicinal combinations are numerous, the list is not complete. For instance, *xìng rén* (apricot kernel), *kǔ xìng rén* (bitter apricot [kernel]), and *bèi mǔ* (fritillaria [bulb]) [*xiàng bèi mǔ* (Zhejiang fritillaria)] are typically used for cough due to external contraction. However, if there is an insufficiency of lung yin with simultaneous symptoms of internal heat, or if the external pathogen has begun to be resolved and yet the phlegmatic cough is not completely resolved, then *nán xìng rén* (southern apricot kernel), [*tián xìng rén* (sweet apricot kernel)], and *chuān bèi mǔ* (Sichuan fritillaria [bulb]) also may be used in combination. [As such] they are rendered in prescriptions as *tián kǔ xìng* and *chuān xiàng bèi*.

Still, one may combine three distinct types of medicinals such as *xìng rén* (apricot kernel), *yì yǐ rén* (coix [seed]), and *bái dòu kòu* (cardamom). Used together these substances diffuse and transform dampness from all three burners. In another area of practice, *shén qū* (medicated leaven), *shān zhā* (crataegus [fruit]), and *mài yá* (barley sprout) are used [in combination] to digest food. They are often burnt and have not been mentioned in the preceding materials.

In summary, the combination of medicinal substances is of major import. If only one aspect is understood and the whys and wherefores are not understood, or if medicinals are simply combined at random, then confusion and needless duplication results.

5. ON THE QUESTIONS OF FREQUENCY AND DOSE IN THE USE OF MEDICINALS

At present there is no standard for the number of medicinals and the dose to be used in prescriptions. There may be as many as twenty ingredients in a prescription, with doses of upwards of several liǎng per ingredient. This practice has produced considerable controversy. I believe that the source of this phenomenon lies in the fact that this [practice] also existed in the past and thus discrepancies have arisen in the way people prescribe today. Nevertheless, there are general criteria for prescription that must be based principally on the pathological condition. These criteria are necessarily of two types: one criterion is that severe conditions require heavy doses and mild conditions require lighter doses. Another criterion is, to the contrary, that a severe condition requires a smaller number of heavier doses, so that its strength is specific and vigorous, while a milder condition requires a larger number of lighter doses, so its strength is dispersed and mild.

The *Nèi Jīng* advocated the use large formulas *[dà fāng]* and small formulas *[xiǎo fāng]*. Quite early on, it proposed:

> If the formula is large then the number of administrations is few, and if it is small then the number of administrations is many — many being nine, and few being two.

It also stated:

> With one sovereign and two ministers, the formulations are considered to be small; [with] two sovereigns, three ministers, and five assistants, formulations are considered to be midsized. With one sovereign, three ministers, and nine assistants, the formulations are considered to be large.

Thus it may be seen that the doses of medicinals in prescriptions has always varied greatly and so cannot be standardized in the clinic.

If we do not proceed from a practical perspective but consider only that more medicinals are more comprehensive and that heavy prescriptions are bolder and more heroic, then not only is the potential of these medicines squandered, but patients also misunderstand [the appropriate principles] and view Chinese medicine as ineffective. Our ancestors have criticized the heavy doses that have appeared in prescriptions. To paraphrase Fāng Guǎng in *Dān Xī Xīn Fǎ Fù Yú:* Zhòngjǐng used no more than three to five ingredients in a prescription, including sovereign, minister, assistant, and envoy. The primary treatment target, the guiding channel entry, and the minute differences in dose were all arranged in the most orderly manner, unlike later generations that employed twenty to thirty ingredients in a prescription.

[Fāng Guǎng] also also cites evidence that Zhū Dānxī established prescriptions modeled on the prescriptions of Zhòngjǐng and used medicinals in a manner that was modeled on that of Lǐ [Dōngyuán]. Stating they were modeled on Zhòngjǐng is indicative of precision in the organization of the prescriptions. Saying that they were modeled on [Lǐ] Dōngyuán's use of medicinals points to his meticulous medicinal combinations. It is generally acknowledged that Lǐ Dōngyuán used a relatively large number of medicinals; nonetheless, his prescriptions were well integrated and not in the least chaotic. As such, they merit emulation. The prescription and the use of medicinals within that prescription are one and the same, and thus are not two separate issues.

It is of primary importance that the rationale be stated first and only then should one consider the actual prescription and medicinals to be used. Otherwise, one's understanding of established prescriptions will be purely mechanical and the medicinals will be thrown together regardless of whether the substances are appropriate or not. Or, if a particular symptom is identified, a particular medicinal will be used in a simplistic treatment. The focal points [necessary for skillful prescribing] will not be grasped and the manner in which all these things should be integrated [in treatment] will not be understood. The former is referred to as having a prescription with no medicinals, and the latter is referred to as having medicinals but no prescription; both must be avoided.

[Lǐ] Dōngyuán's prescriptions were not like this. He crafted famous prescriptions for the spleen and stomach, using with admiration Zhāng Jiégǔ's reliance on Zhāng Zhòngjǐng's prescription *Zhǐ Zhù Tāng* (Unripe Bitter Orange and Ovate Atractylodes Decoction), which [Lǐ Dōngyuán] adapted to produce *Zhǐ Zhù Wán* (Unripe Bitter Orange and Ovate Atractylodes Pill). He recognized that the dose of *bái zhú* (ovate atractylodes [root]) should be double that of *zhǐ ké* (bitter orange) – one being supplementing and one being draining, one relaxing and one urgent – and he understood that they were used differently. Nevertheless, when used clinically *bàn xià* (pinellia [tuber]) is added [and this yields *Bàn Xià Zhǐ Zhù Wán* (Pinella, Unripe Bitter Orange, and Ovate Atractylodes Pill)]. *Jú hóng* (red tangerine peel) may be added [and this yields *Jú Hóng Zhǐ Zhù Wán* (Red Tangerine Peel, Unripe Bitter Orange, and Ovate Atractylodes Pill)]. *Shén qū* (medicated leaven), *mài yá* (barley sprout), and *gǔ yá* (rice sprout) may be added [and this yields *Qū Niè Zhǐ Zhù Wán* (Medicated Leaven, Barley Sprout, Unripe Bitter Orange, and Ovate Atractylodes Pill)]. *Huáng lián* (coptis [root]), *huáng qín* (scutellaria [root]), *dà huáng* (rhubarb), *jú hóng* (red tangerine peel), and *shén qū* (medicated leaven) may also be added [and this makes *Sān Huáng Zhǐ Zhú Wán* (Three Yellows Bitter Orange and Ovate Atractylodes Pill)].

None of these modifications may be applied rigidly.

Moreover, in the sweet, warm, heat-clearing prescription *Bǔ Zhōng Yì Qì Tāng* (Center-Supplementing Qi-Boosting Decoction) used in cases of insufficiency of spleen-stomach, sweet was originally preferred and bitter avoided, supplementation was preferred and contraction avoided, warm was preferred and cold avoided, freeing was preferred and girdling avoided, upbearing was preferred and downbearing avoided, dry was preferred and damp was avoided. Therefore, *huáng qí* (astragalus [root]), *rén shēn* (ginseng), and *gān cǎo* (licorice [root]) were used to supplement the qi. *Shēng má* (cimicifuga [root]) and *chái hú* (bupleurum [root]) were used to upbear the yang. *Dāng guī* (tangkuei) harmonized the generation of blood. *Bái zhú* (ovate atractylodes [root]) benefited the rectification of dampness and *qīng pí* (unripe tangerine peel) regulated the coursing of qi. Although there are a relatively large number of ingredients, the objectives are clear, the primary and secondary goals are clearly delineated, and the combinations are tightly knit. Moreover, out of this have come more than twenty modifications, employing a variety of medicinal substances including:

fáng fēng	ledebouriella [root]
qiāng huó	notopterygium [root]
qīng pí	unripe tangerine peel
mù xiāng	saussurea [root]
bái dòu kòu	cardamom
bīn láng	areca [nut]
bái sháo yào	white peony [root]
chuān xiōng	ligusticum [root]
bàn xià	pinellia [tuber]
fù zǐ	aconite [accessory tuber]
huáng lián	coptis [root]
mài mén dōng	ophiopogon [tuber]
wǔ wèi zǐ	schisandra [berry]

Prescription doses here are one qián each and, if the illness is severe, more is administered, because it is said, "establish the dose according to treatment."

This small example illustrates the methods our ancestors employed in prescribing formulas and prescriptions. Naturally, however, we need not, nor is it appropriate, to cleave to the conventions of the ancients.

In summary, we can say that the essential issue is that of getting an appropriate grasp on dosage in prescribing medicinals. I believe that while there are definite criteria [for these decisions], they are not rigidly fixed. In terms of general disease patterns, medicinal prescriptions will often include from fifteen or sixteen ingredients up to more than twenty ingredients. Upward of one liǎng of *huáng qí* (astragalus [root]) and *fù zǐ* (aconite [accessory tuber]) may be used, while *lián qiáo* (forsythia [fruit]), *sāng yè* (mulberry leaf), *jú huā* (chrysanthemum [flower]), *jīng jiè* (schizonepeta), and *fáng fēng* (ledebouriella [root]) may be used in doses of up to three or four qián. It seems to me that this is unnecessary.

6. PRESCRIPTION FORMAT

I have discussed the format of Chinese medical prescriptions time and again and there are likely some of you who do not understand why this is [the case], or have mistaken this as a doctrinaire approach. Actually, I believe that a prescription should have a fixed format, although in the past it has been said that such a fixed format contains just the same old stuff. Nonetheless, prescription format is part of a fine tradition and its preservation is still appropriate. For example, in the past prescriptions were written in vertical lines from right to left, while today, the words are written sideways from left to right. These are only the obvious differences.

In the past, the arrangement of the medicinal substances was divided into three lines, with three rows to a line. Its sequence was that the first row of each of the three lines was written first, followed next by the second [row], and then the final one. If there was a medicinal guide, it was to be written on the fourth line, one character beneath the top row. In this way the sovereign medicinals were written first, then the ministerial, assistant, and envoy medicinals were written in sequence such that primary and secondary medicinals were clearly divided.

In the case of horizontal script I believe that three ingredients should be written in the first line, followed successively in the second and third lines, as this is also quite distinct and, moreover, when there are a large number of ingredients, a fourth or fifth line may be appended as convenient. It must be pointed out that medicinals generally have primary and secondary roles in treatment and those of principal importance are written first, followed by those of secondary importance. This approach not only reflects the orientation of the therapy, but is also orderly.

Old Style Prescription				
	3	2	1	Sovereign
	6	5	4	Minister
10	9	8	7	Envoy

New Style Prescription				
	1	2	3	Sovereign
	4	5	6	Minister
	7	8	9	Envoy
10				Guide

Medicinal combinations should also be clear at a glance. For example, when *Yín Qiào Sǎn* (Lonicera and Forsythia Powder) is used, *jīn yín huā* (lonicera [flower]) and *lián qiáo* (forsythia [fruit]) are most often written first. It is my opinion that in using *Yín Qiào Sǎn* in warm disorders one may naturally lead off with *jīn yín huā* (lonicera [flower]) and *lián qiáo* (forsythia [fruit]). Yet, whether or not *lián qiáo* is a sovereign medicinal merits consideration. If *lián qiáo* is the designated or sovereign, then what is the ministerial medicinal?

It is my opinion that for *Yín Qiào Săn* the primary disorder is wind-warm, and wind-warm is a disorder resulting from an external contraction. External pathogens in the first stage should all be treated by resolving the exterior, and *Yín Qiào Săn* is based upon the premise [that]: "in the case of wind environmental repletion, treat with acrid cool medicinals assisted by bitter sweet." This is referred to as "acrid cool methods for resolving the surface." In this way, the organization of the prescription would make the wind coursing medicinals, *dòu chǐ* (fermented soybean), *jīng jiè suì* (schizonepeta spike), and *bò hé* (mint) sovereign. *Jīn yín huā* (lonicera [flower]), *lián qiáo* (forsythia [fruit]), and *zhú yè* (black bamboo leaf) are used to address the pathogenic warm factor. Because the pathogen is in the lung, *niú bàng zǐ* (arctium [seed]) and *jié gěng* (platycodon [root]) are used to open and diffuse the upper burner. Finally, the addition of sweet *gān căo* (licorice [root]) clears heat and resolves toxins, while fresh *lú gēn* (phragmites [root]) clears heat, arrests thirst, and harmonizes the entire preparation when it is decocted. In light of this arrangement, the prescription is appropriate.

However, if resolving the exterior is primary, then why use medicinals for clearing heat to name the prescription? This redresses the mistaken use prevalent at the time [this prescription was conceived] of using acrid warm diaphoretic measures to treat warm disorders.[8] This is not to suggest that in treating wind heat disorders, the surface need not be resolved as long as the heat is cleared. Naturally, such an interpretation may only be acquired by studying the prescription. Nevertheless, this rationale must be understood when prescribing, so that we will be skillful and not depart in a muddled direction by transposing the surface resolving medicinals in a mixed-up and confused manner.

In the past, the way in which the names of medicinals were recorded in a prescription differed from how they were written in pharmacopias. Some prescriptions included the place of origin, and some denoted the degree of quality, as well as the method of drug processing. This is what is called "prescription terminology" *[chù fāng yǒu míng]*. Why is it important to write prescriptions in this manner? The place of origin is of principal concern for the maximization of therapeutic effect. Therefore, the pharmacist [filling the prescription] will advertise his use of a genuine [high quality] medicine to appeal to his market.

Since there is now a national monopoly on the purchase and marketing of today's medicinal products and they are honestly sold at reduced prices, the trust of the masses was gained early. Therefore, I think that the wording regarding the place of production and methodology of preparation can now be economized. Nevertheless, the majority [of practitioners] pay no attention [to this information] and are in the habit of referencing the nomenclature of pharmacopoeias. For example, there are two types of *xìng rén* (apricot kernel): sweet *[tián]* and bitter *[kŭ]*, and when used, the skin may be removed and the tip broken away. *Kŭ xìng rén* (bitter apricot kernel) is generally used in prescriptions and, therefore, is written *"xìng rén"* [guāng xìng rén, "naked," or "simple" apricot kernel]. If the skin must be left on, then it is written as *dài pí xìng* ["clothed" or "belted"

[8]Trans: This is a reference to what Qin considered mistaken procedures proposed during the Qing dynasty.

apricot kernel]. [On the other hand,] these days [often] only the two words "apricot kernel" *[xìng rén]* are written, which is a rather oversimplified practice. There are many other examples, for instance, *bèi mǔ* (fritillaria [bulb]) may be *xiàng bèi mǔ* (Zhejiang fritillaria [bulb]), or *chuān bèi mǔ* (Sichuan fritillaria [bulb]), but is [often] written only as *bèi mǔ*. *Tǔ niú xī* (native achyranthes [root]) may be *huái niú xī* (achyranthes [root]) or *chuān niú xī* (cyathula [root]) but is written only as *niú xī*. *Shí gāo* (gypsum) also may be used crude *[shēng]* or cooked *[shóu]* but is written only as *shí gāo*. *Bàn xià* (pinellia [tuber]) may be used in both raw or prepared forms. Of the various prepared forms there is *jiāng bàn xià* (ginger[-processed] pinellia [tuber]), *qīng bàn xià* (purified pinellia), and *zhú lì bàn xià* (bamboo sap pinellia [tuber]), which are all written only as *bàn xià*.

All these are issues [to consider]. We must understand that the specific varieties of Chinese medicinals and their medicinal preparation are issues of fundamental importance, however, such differences in nomenclature may be ignored based [only on one's certain knowledge of] what is in [local] supply. For instance, if we simply write *shí gāo* (gypsum), some places [only] have it on-hand raw, and some places [only] have it on-hand prepared, and so there may be great discrepancies in its efficacy. For this reason, I advocate that some principal medicinal substances that vary in efficacy because of their location or origin [of production] are best written as more than a single word. One should not be unnecessarily succinct.

Up to now [physicians have often used] pseudonymous names for medicinals. For instance, *jīn yín huā* (lonicera [flower]) is sometimes written as "*èr bǎo huā*" and "*shuāng huā*," and *pàng dà hài* (sterculia) is sometimes written as "*ān nán zǐ*." *Bīn láng* (areca [nut]) is sometimes written as as "*hǎi nán ǎi*." One must exercise restraint in showing off the extent of one's knowledge and this must be a reform within today's society.

In composing prescriptions to be filled by a pharmacy, the name of the medicinal and the dose must be neat and clear, and the script must not be sloppy. Simplified characters should be in accordance with the State Department publication, *"Notice on Writing Prescriptions with Simplified Characters" ["Hàn Zì Jiǎn Huà Fāng Àn"]* and should not be some fabrication [of one's own invention]. While these requirements seem harsh, nevertheless, unforseen errors and mishaps will be avoided [if this practice is followed]. While it will be slow in the beginning, once we are practiced in this convention it will not require much effort.[9]

In summary, attention must be paid to the format of the prescription, because not only is there an issue of raising one's professional level but also of assisting the pharmacies in filling prescriptions. Everything must be in the service of the people and everything must benefit the peoples' interest. Particularly [with a view toward] the party's development of high level Chinese medical practitioners, this fine tradition should be carried on because it is a good model.

(February 1962)

---

[9]Trans: This reflects something of the difficulties Chinese health authorities faced in their attempt to develop a standard practice of T.C.M. as regards local and individual practices.

CHINESE MEDICAL THERAPY FOR ABATING FEVER

Translator's Introduction

The symptom of fever may be conceptualized in several ways. It may be understood within the context of a discrimination of patterns of internal origin, such as yin vacuity or damp heat, or it may be understood within the context of patterns of external origin, such as the *Shāng Hán* six level patterns, triple burner patterns, or the *Wēn Bìng* four aspect patterns. In studying this essay, the reader should remember that these frameworks for discussing the invasion of external pathogens may also be more simply used as convenient landmarks for labeling the depth and location of an illness, that is, for the "patholocale" as Qin describes it. This is true even when the concept of external invasion is largely irrelevant and, in fact, this assumption is one of the pillars of the Japanese adaptation of internal medicine known as *Kanpo Yaku.*

It is a distinct characteristic of modern T.C.M. that the six levels and four aspects are used primarily as points of reference rather than thought of as stages of a progession. While they may be implied within the context of the *Shāng Hán* six levels, the related treatment methods are often not strictly part of that system. For instance, a patient with fever alternating with chills accompanied by thoracocostal fullness, nausea, a bitter taste in the mouth, and a wiry pulse would be diagnosed as suffering from a *shào yáng* pattern and the guiding principle would be *xiǎo chái hú tāng* (Minor Bupleurum Decoction). However, the specific treatment formula of "abating fever by harmonization and resolution" is one of the later theoretical additions to the *Shāng Hán* system that is characteristic of modern T.C.M.

It has been my experience that most modern Chinese T.C.M. practitioners think in terms of the six levels or four aspects only when it is convenient for conceptualizing a problem within the general T.C.M. framework. While they are invariably well versed in these models of illness, their most basic operating system is that of pattern identification associated with the viscera and bowels. Furthermore, the various levels and aspects are generally utilized as reference points for the location and depth of the illness. For instance, while a pathogenic factor is likely to be implicit in most references to "*tài yáng* levels" or the "protective aspect," references to the "*shào yīn* level" or the "constructive and blood aspects" explicitly denote the relative physical level of an illness and its attendant symptoms. Today such references may be made totally without reference to an externally invading pathogenic factor. In fact, in China the very notion of actual pathogen progression from the *tài yáng* down to the *shào yīn* has been discarded by many practitioners as clinically irrelevant. While the levels and aspects themselves may be thought to have some basis in clinical reality, many feel that the notion of an orderly progression from one to another does not. In sum, while they recognize the validity or utility of the clinical observations that are the foundation of the classical theory, they do not recognize the theory itself as valid. Such a perspective naturally produces a conceptually segmented model of illness.

Qin Bowei's discussion of fever is organized around the treatment methods indicated in addressing sixteen of the most common fever patterns. As such his thought characterizes a distinctly T.C.M. approach to this material. In this, T.C.M. is an umbrella paradigm under which every model is subsumed, including the six levels, the four aspects, and the triple burner patterns. This is evident in all of Qin's writings. His ideas are presented not within the context of any single systematic progression of illness but instead in a manner much more akin to the format of prescription manuals and, to a lesser extent, pharmacopia. The general progression is from the outside inward, however it does not follow conventions related to any specific pathological process.

Qin Bowei's arrangement of the yang levels in the six level progression will seem unusual to Western-trained readers. While this progression is most often taught as proceeding from *tài yáng* to *shào yáng* to *yáng míng*, Qin Bowei felt that an ordering from *tài yáng*, to *yáng míng* and then *shào yang* was of greater clinical utility. In fact, in his work this is the "correct" order. He saw the *shào yáng* as the pivot between the inside and outside of the body. In this context, "inside" denotes the yin viscera as opposed to the yang bowels on the "outside." His examples of *má huáng* (ephedra), *gé gēn* (pueraria [root]), and *chái hú* (bupleurum [root]), corresponding to the *tài yáng*, *yáng míng,* and *shào yáng* respectively, relate to the use of these medicinals as guides for the overall prescription. In other words, pueraria guides the effect of a formula to the *yáng míng* level.

CHINESE MEDICAL THERAPY FOR ABATING FEVER

Fevers are an obvious symptom that are commonly encountered [in clinical practice]. Because their etiology is complex, they involve many illness categories. In clinical practice fevers may be a primary complaint by a patient during an initial examination and, especially at the initial onset, a precise diagnosis of a fever may be quite problematic. Chinese medicine utilizes the methodology of pattern identification and treatment, discriminating among variations in the morphology of the fever and its associated symptoms, while simultaneously differentiating etiologies and the locality of the disease. From this, the course of the illness and the development of the situation can be evaluated to promote the timely execution of the appropriate therapies.

All of this is documented in complete detail in the [Chinese] medical literature. Based simply on my own clinical experience, it is evident to me that Chinese medicine approaches the treatment of fever in a systematic manner. This means that as far as prescription methods for abating fevers are concerned, the medicine of our homeland contains an integrated therapeutic system, which appears to be even more comprehensive than that of modern Western medicine. At present, I believe that I have a preliminary understanding of the Chinese medical treatment of fevers and would like to introduce an outline of that understanding. This narration is incomplete and also insufficiently detailed. The guiding prescriptions I have provided are only cited for illustrative purposes and are not formulas that have special effects for the treatment of fevers. If this discussion should veer off in an inappropriate direction, I hope everyone will be generous with criticism!

1. Methods for Abating Fever by Diaphoresis

Diaphoretic substances act to dissipate the body temperature, thus lowering an elevated body temperature and, in this regard, Chinese and Western medicine hold identical points of view. Chinese medicine posits that methods for abating fever by diaphoresis are indicated for fevers that are due to the contraction of an external pathogen at the exterior of the body. Febrile illnesses due to external pathogens on the exterior are referred to as "exterior patterns." Because diaphoresis treats exterior heat, it is also referred to as "resolving the exterior." External pathogens vary in type and nature, and diaphoresis is merely a basic treatment method. Specific applications must be based on a diagnosis of the type of external pathogens present. Then, appropriate medicinals may be selected from the category for resolving the exterior.

Differentiation of the two major categories of diaphoresis, acrid warm diaphoresis and acrid cool diaphoresis, is of primary importance. It should be understood that in applying diaphoresis, medicinals possessed of an acrid taste are the principal component and are combined in therapy with substances of a warm or cool nature. Acrid warm medicinals are mostly used for contractions of wind-cold, while acrid and cool medicinals are mostly used for wind-heat. Patterns of wind-cold and wind-heat are differentiated in this way: in the former there will be fever and aversion to cold, no desire to remove one's clothing, dry skin, adiaphoresis, headache and occipital tension, soreness and pain of the muscles and articulations of the entire body, a thin white or thick slimy tongue moss, and a floating, tense, and rapid pulse. In the latter condition of wind-heat there will be fever and aversion to wind, a sensation of pressure in the head, spontaneous sweating, dry mouth, a thin slimy or yellow-colored tongue moss, and a pulse that is slippery and rapid or that is bilaterally large only in the cubit position.

Regardless of whether it is wind-cold or wind-heat, all fevers fall within the category of external afflictions and are often accompanied by symptoms of bronchial infection, such as scratchy throat, cough, nasal obstruction, and drainage.   Nonetheless, wind-heat and wind-cold patterns differ in severity. [In cases of the usually more common wind-heat pattern] the nasal orifices commonly contract heat, phlegm is difficult to expectorate, or there is throat pain.

Acrid warm diaphoretic formulas are exemplified by the following prescriptions:

Má Huáng Tāng (Ephedra Decoction)	
Zhāng Zhòngjǐng's prescription	
má huáng	ephedra
guì zhī	cinnamon twig
xìng rén	apricot kernel
gān cǎo	licorice [root]

Xiāng Sū Yǐn (Cyperus and Perilla Beverage)	
from *Hé Jì Jú Fāng*	
zǐ sū yè	perilla leaf
xiāng fù zǐ	cyperus [root]
chén pí	tangerine peel
gān cǎo	licorice [root]
shēng jiāng	fresh ginger
xiè bái	Chinese chive [bulb]

Acrid cool diaphoretic formulas are exemplified by the following prescriptions:

Yín Qiào Sǎn (Lonicera and Forsythia Decoction)	
Wú Jútōng's prescription	
jīn yín huā	lonicera [flower]
lián qiáo	forsythia [fruit]
bò hé	mint
jīng jiè suì	schizonepeta spike
jié gěng	platycodon [root]
dòu chǐ	fermented soybean
niú bàng zǐ	arctium [seed]
zhú yè black	bamboo leaf
gān cǎo	licorice [root]
lú gēn	phragmites [root]

Sāng Jú Yǐn (Mulberry Leaf and Chrysanthemum Beverage)	
Wú Jútōng's prescription	
sāng yè	mulberry leaf
jú huā	chrysanthemum [flower]
bò hé	mint
xìng rén	apricot kernel
lián qiáo	forsythia [fruit]
jié gěng	platycodon [root]
gān cǎo	licorice [root]
lú gēn	(phragmites [root])

These formulations are not comprised of only diaphoretics that are acrid and warm or acrid and cool but also incorporate substances for clearing heat, suppressing cough, and clearing the head and eyes. Therefore, when diaphoresis has occurred and the symptoms have dissipated, there will be a speedy return to health. Moreover, in terms of medicinals for resolving toxins and harmonizing the stomach, these should never have side effects on the stomach and will rarely cause poor digestion and nausea, nor will they cause the symptoms of tinnitus, edematous swelling, and urticaria.

Other than external pathogens such as wind-cold and wind-heat, we commonly encounter pathogens such as dampness, summerheat, and autumn dryness. Because the nature of dampness tends to be cold and the nature of summerheat and dryness tends to be hot, the medication to be selected for each of these conditions differs. External dampness is a result of the contraction of pathogens of fog and dew, with symptoms of fever, sensation of pressure in the head as if it were wrapped, thoracic oppression, and vexation soreness in the body. {The following prescription is] indicated:

Shén Zhú Sǎn (Wondrous Atractylodes Powder)	
Tài Wúfāng's prescription	
cāng zhú	atractylodes [root]
tǔ huò xiāng	agastache
hòu pò	magnolia bark
chén pí	tangerine peel
shí chāng pú	acorus [root]
gān cǎo	licorice [root]
jiāng	ginger
suān zǎo rén	spiny jujube [kernel]

The symptoms of contraction of summerheat are steaming fever in the flesh, headache and heaviness of the head, lassitude, and vexation thirst. [The following prescription is] indicated:

Modified *Xiāng Rú Yǐn* (Elsholtsia Powder)	
from *Hé Jì Jú Fāng*	
xiāng róu	elsholtzia
huáng lián	coptis [root]
dòu chǐ	fermented soybean
hòu pò	magnolia bark

Autumnal dryness is a seasonal illness related to the autumn season and patients suffer from a slight fever, sensation of baking heat in the nostrils, dry cough, and chapped lips with a dry mouth. [The following prescription is] indicated:

Sāng Xīng Tāng (Mulberry Leaf and Apricot Kernel Decoction)	
Wú Jútōng's prescription	
sāng yè	mulberry leaf
xìng rén	apricot kernel
hēi dà dòu	black soybean
běi shā shēn	glehnia [root]
shān zhī pí	gardenia husk
lí pí	pear peel
xiàng bèi mǔ	Zhejiang fritillaria [bulb]

External pathogens may cause a variety of feverish illnesses; for instance, mumps resulting in parotitis with chills and fever, and pressing pain anterior and posterior to the ear; throat moth resulting in tonsillitis with chills and fever, reddening of the eyes, tearing of the eyes on exposure to the wind, gingival swelling resulting in peridontitis with chills and fever, and swelling and distension in the gums resulting in pain and suppuration. The formulas of choice are [as follows:]

Chái Hú Gě Gēn Tāng (Bupleurum and Pueraria Decoction)	
Yī Zōngjīn's prescription	
chái hú	bupleurum [root]
gé gēn	pueraria [root]
huáng qín	scutellaria [root]
shí gāo	gypsum
tiān huā fěn	trichosanthes [root]
niú bàng zǐ	arctium [seed]
jīn yín huā	lonicera [flower]
jié gěng	platycodon [root]
gān cǎo	licorice [root]
shēng má	cimicifuga [root]

Gān Jié Shè Gān Tāng (Licorice, Platycodon, and Belamcanda Decoction)	
from *Shěng Shì Zhūn Shēng Shū*	
gān cǎo	licorice [root]
jié gěng	platycodon [root]
wū shàn	belamcanda [root]
shān dòu gēn	bushy sophora [root]
lián qiáo	forsythia [fruit]
fáng fēng	ledebouriella [root]
jīng jiè suì	schizonepeta spike
xuán shēn	scrophularia [root]
niú bàng zǐ	arctium [seed]
zhú yè	black bamboo leaf

Xī Gān Sǎn (Liver-Washing Powder)	
from *Shěng Shì Yáo Hán*	
dāng guī	tangkuei
chuān xiōng	ligusticum [root]
bò hé	mint
xiān dì huáng	fresh raw rehmannia [root]
qiāng huó	notopterygium [root]
shān zhī zǐ	gardenia [fruit]
fáng fēng	ledebouriella [root]
dà huáng	rhubarb
lóng dǎn	gentian [root]
gān cǎo	licorice [root]

Xiè Huáng Sǎn (Yellow-Draining Powder)	
from Qián Yǐ's prescription	
fáng fēng	ledebouriella [root]
tǔ huò xiāng	agastache
shān zhī zǐ	gardenia [fruit]
shí gāo	gypsum
gān cǎo	licorice [root]

[These prescriptions] are appropriate for use based on variations in the symptoms and location of the illness.

Diaphoretic prescriptions for the febrile patterns mentioned above are quite extensive [in number], and although they are divided into classes of acrid warm and acrid cool, these are both large categories in and of themselves. Since the nature of the symptom presentation for external pathogens varies, methods such as clearing heat, analgesia, and resolving toxins are also combined with acrid cool or acrid warm diaphoresis, and whenever the organization of the prescription is based on modulations within the illness, the composition of the prescription will also be complex.[1] Beyond the capacity of diaphoretics to abate fever, they may also injure the fluids and induce unchecked diaphoresis, creating a variety of pathological changes with symptoms of yang collapse vacuity desertion and so forth. Therefore, even more than administering appropriate doses [of the medicinals composing] formulas, particular caution should be exercised in vacuity symptom patterns or for patients with vacuous constitutions.

2. Methods for Abating Fever by Regulation and Harmonization of the Constructive and the Defensive

Simply put, the meaning of harmonization and regulation of the constructive and defensive is the regulation of any imbalances within the qi and blood. The constructive blood is internal, while the defensive qi is external. If a wind pathogen is contracted in the defensive aspect, with fever in the skin and muscle, nasal congestion, noisy respiration, and spontaneous perspiration, this takes the form of weakness of the constructive and strength of the defensive. In this situation the wind pathogen must be expelled through the harmonization of the qi and blood. Therefore, the regulation and harmonization of the constructive and defensive is in reality a method for resolving the exterior, and typically used are prescriptions such as:

Guì Zhī Tāng (Cinnamon Twig Decoction)	
Zhāng Zhòngjǐng's prescription	
guì zhī	cinnamon twig
bái sháo yào	white peony [root]
gān cǎo	licorice [root]
jiāng	ginger
dà zǎo	jujube [fruit]

Nevertheless, the principle of regulation and harmonization of the constructive and defensive is not the same as that of diaphoresis.

Guì Zhī Tāng (Cinnamon Twig Decoction) uses *guì zhī* (cinnamon twig) to dispel wind and *bái sháo yào* (white peony [root]) to harmonize the blood. It uses *shēng jiāng* (fresh ginger) to promote the exterior and *dà zǎo* (jujube [fruit]) to supplement the middle.

---

[1]Trans: "Modulations" are changes of the herbs in a prescription relative to the presenting illness. If the variations of the illness are complex, the formula will be complex.

Although it is referred to as a diaphoretic prescription, it obviously differs from prescriptions that specifically abate fever by diaphoresis. I believe that regulating and harmonizing the constructive and defensive supports bodily function in expelling external pathogens and the symptoms for which it is appropriate are aversion to cold and aversion to wind and fever. The pulse is floating and slow or floating in the cun position and weak in the cubit position. Following administration of Cinnamon Twig Decoction, the patient should drink hot thin gruel, cover themselves with bed clothing, and lie down so as to assist the diaphoresis.

The wind-coursing and fever-abating function of *Guì Zhī Tāng* (Cinnamon Twig Decoction) is different from diaphoretic prescriptions in general, and therefore Cinnamon Twig Decoction is not indicated for exterior repletion patterns with adiaphoresis, and the doses of the various ingredients should also reflect this [fact]. In Cinnamon Twig Decoction the doses of cinnamon twig and white peony [root] are equal in the source prescription. If the amount of cinnamon twig used is greater than that of white peony [root], or if the dose of white peony [root] exceeds that of cinnamon twig, the condition [for which the formula is] indicated will be quite different. Also, because Cinnamon Twig Decoction is able to regulate and harmonize the constructive and the defensive aspects, if modified it is also capable of treating vacuity patterns such as in [its permutations] *Huáng Qí Jiàn Zhōng Tāng* (Astragalus Center-Fortifying Decoction), *Xiǎo Jiàng Zhōng Tāng* (Minor Center-Fortifying Decoction), and others. This is a distinguishing feature of this prescription.

3. METHODS FOR ABATING FEVER BY CLEARING THE STOMACH

If an exterior affliction accompanied by fever is unresolved, then the pathogen may gradually move deeper, presenting as symptoms of sustained high fever, an aversion to heat rather than aversion to cold, a fever that increases in severity in the afternoon, copious perspiration, thirst with an increased intake of fluids, a thin yellow tongue coat and a flooding, large, and rapid pulse. This is referred to in Chinese medicine as a *yáng míng* channel pattern. *Yáng míng* pertains to the stomach channel and at this point diaphoretic methods cannot be mistakenly employed, because this will produce the serious condition of yang desertion and yin exhaustion. Neither can one nourish the yin alone, because this promotes the pathological changes of excessive yin, which further inhibits the yang. Thus the use of slightly acrid, sweet, cold, stomach-clearing methods is indicated through the use of prescriptions such as:

Bái Hǔ Tāng (White Tiger Decoction)	
Zhāng Zhòngjǐng's prescription	
shí gāo	gypsum
zhī mǔ	anemarrhena [root]
gān cǎo	licorice [root]
gǔ yá	rice sprout

On the one hand, [this prescription] preserves the fluids, and, on the other hand, [it] outthrusts and drains heat pathogens from the exterior muscles. This variety of symptom pattern is quite often seen in the course of [both] injury by cold and warm illness. Since it is still hoped that the pathogen will be expelled from the exterior, diaphoresis therefore naturally occurs following administration of the medicine, and this most often forces out the foul qi. At this stage of the illness, Chinese medicine does not advocate the use of ice bags or cold drinks because such methods conflict with the therapeutic methods described above and should thus be avoided.

In the similar category of internal heat with cardiac vexation and delirium, sweet and cold medicinals are insufficient to treat them, thus bitter cold methods are indicated with prescriptions such as:

Dà Huáng Huáng Lián Xiè Xīn Tāng (Rhubarb and Coptis Heart-Draining Decoction)	
Zhāng Zhòngjǐng's prescription	
dà huáng	rhubarb
huáng lián	coptis [root]

or

Huáng Lián Jiě Dú Tāng (Coptis Toxin-Resolving Decoction)	
Cuī Shìfāng's prescription	
huáng lián	coptis [root]
huáng qín	scutellaria [root]
huáng bǎi	phellodendron [bark]
shān zhī zǐ	gardenia [fruit]

I believe that sweet cold methods and bitter cold methods are completely different and that their intent is also different. Nevertheless, both have strong heat-clearing and toxin-resolving functions. The forte of sweet cold methods for abating fever is that they expel the pathogen by diaphoresis, while restricting the production of a higher body temperature and protecting against a desiccation of fluids. Bitter cold formulas drain the pathogen and, in general, the spirit symptoms then gradually diminish or disappear. This is an excellent example of properly [practiced] Chinese medicine first treating the cause of the illness and thus overcoming the main symptoms.[2]

4. METHODS FOR ABATING FEVER BY FREEING THE STOOL

An exuberance of heat in the stomach will almost certainly injure the fluids of the water aspect. This also influences the intestines toward an obstructive binding of the stools. In this case, not only is the fever unabated but the fever also steams, increasing rather than diminishing, intensifying in the afternoon. There is vexation agitation, clouded spirit and delirium, and yellow, slimy, and coarse or black and thorny tongue and moss. Urgent administration of [the following] prescription to free and disinhibit the stools is indicated:

---

[2]Trans: The use of medicinals that are sweet and cold clear heat by diaphoresis and protect the fluids. The use of medicinals that are bitter and cold focus on draining the pathogen. With the pathogen thus eliminated the symptoms resolve on their own.

Dà Chéng Qì Tāng (Major Qi-Infusing Decoction)	
Zhāng Zhòngjǐng's prescription	
dà huáng	rhubarb
máng xiāo	mirabilite
zhǐ shí	unripe bitter orange
hòu pò	magnolia bark

Such a drastic method is called for in this situation. [In Chinese medical writing] this is likened to removing the wood from the furnace, thus, naturally, the water is not boiled away. *Dà Chéng Qì Tāng* (Major Qi-Infusing Decoction) is a formula for heavy precipitation, and thus symptoms of agitation, repletion and strength, and hardness and fullness should be present. There will be abdominal distension and pain upon palpation; thus this prescription may be used when there is definitely dry excrement in the intestines. If there is an insufficiency of fluids, this is like a boat with no water, and rather than using methods for pushing the stools out, the prescription is assisted by methods for moistening the intestines.[3] [A prescription representative of this method is:]

Pí Yuē Má Rén Wán (Straitened Spleen Hemp Seed Pill)	
Zhāng Zhòngjǐng's prescription	
huǒ má rén	hemp seed
bái sháo yào	white peony [root]
xìng rén	apricot kernel
dà huáng	rhubarb
zhǐ shí	unripe bitter orange
hòu pò	magnolia bark

Also, if there has been a severe injury to the fluids, the internal administration of draining formulas is unacceptable; however, topical conducting methods may be used. Formerly, *Mì Qiān* (Thickened Honey Enema) Zhāng Zhòngjǐng's prescription containing *liàn mì* (processed honey) and *zào jiá* (gleditsia [fruit]), or *Zhū Dǎn Zhē* (Pig's Bile Sap), Zhāng Zhòngjǐng's prescription containing *zhū dǎn gāo* (pig's bile) and *cù* (vinegar), was used in a manner similar to [how we now use] glycerine suppositories and intestinal irrigation. Nevertheless, in warm illness there may be excessive desiccation of the yin aspect, or a simple vacuity of the patient's yin fluids, so not only are draining formulas contraindicated, but external conducting methods also cannot be used casually. Therefore, in later ages, *Zēng Yè Tāng* (Humor-Increasing Decoction), Wú Jútōng's prescription containing *xuán shēn* (scrophularia [root]), *mài mén dōng* (ophiopogon [tuber]), and *xiān dì huáng* (fresh raw rehmannia [root]) was composed. Supplementing medicinals form the base of this prescription, although it makes use of draining medicinals to eliminate repletion while protecting against vacuity, and this has direct clinical importance.

It is my belief that in terms of general medicinals for freeing the stool, some modern [Western biomedical] prescriptions are superior to herbal medicinals and substitutions may be considered. Nevertheless, in draining formulas for fever patterns one must simultaneously utilize methods for clearing heat, resolving toxins, protecting the yin and engendering fluids. Given the variables involved in the treatment of this condition, draining formulas cannot be discussed in general terms.

---

[3]Trans: "assisted" here is the character for the assisting medicinal in the organization of a prescription. Thus the bowels are assisted by the assisting medicinal in the prescription.

5. METHODS FOR ABATING FEVER BY PROMOTING EJECTION

If there is fever and cardiac vexation, or late stage fever with subcardiac binding accumulation and pain, then ejection methods may be used, incorporating prescriptions such as *Zhī Zǐ Chǐ Tāng* (Gardenia and Fermented Soybean Decoction), Zhāng Zhòngjǐng's prescription containing *shān zhī zǐ* (gardenia [fruit]) and *dòu chǐ* (fermented soybean). With the administration of these formulas there will be slight vomiting.

Our ancestors treated illnesses of a febrile nature with the three major methods of diaphoresis, emesis, and precipitation. In modern times, however, the use of emesis is relatively rare. This may be due to the fact that ejection is more often than not unpleasant for the patient and, in weakened patients, as soon as emesis is induced, there is frequently diaphoresis, rough breathing and an actual increase in the pathological changes. Although it is clear that ejection methods are utilized for dispersion of the cumulative binding of pathogenic heat in the upper burner, it is actually a shortcut to clearing a surplus [or repletion condition in general]. If one is adverse to ejection methods, one may make alternate use of methods for downbearing and precipitation. However, this approach is also capable of inducing counterflow and the pathological changes produced are unpredictable. Our ancestors had important parameters for determining when diaphoresis, precipitation, or emesis were indicated and when they were not. In general, these were based on observation of the appropriate symptoms.

6. METHODS FOR ABATING FEVER BY HARMONIZATION AND RESOLUTION

In the midst of a febrile pattern there may be sudden chills and sudden fever, which will alternate several times in the course of a day in a manner similar to malarial illness but which is not malarial illness. This is called alternating chills and fever *[hán rè wǎng lái]*. The location of the illness is not on the exterior, yet it is also not in the interior. Rather, it is located in the *shào yáng* channel, being half exterior and half interior. Because of this, neither diaphoresis nor precipitation is appropriate; instead, harmonizing prescription methods are indicated. Alternating fever and chills are a characteristic of *shào yáng* illnesses, yet they are accompanied by thoracocostal pi fullness, cardiac vexation and nausea, bitter taste in the mouth, visual dizziness, deafness,[4] and a wiry pulse. The primary prescription to calm the interior and resist foreign aggression is:

Xiǎo Chái Hú Tāng (Minor Bupleurum Decoction)	
Zhāng Zhòngjǐng's prescription	
chái hú	bupleurum [root]
huáng qín	scutellaria [root]
rén shēn	ginseng
bàn xià	pinellia [tuber]
gān cǎo	licorice [root]
jiāng	ginger
dà zǎo	jujube [fruit]

[4]Trans: The pathogen can be mediated into the ear through the *shào yáng* vessel of the gallbladder and triple burner channels. This deafness due to a repletion pathogen is distinct from deafness due to kidney vacuity.

Because *shào yáng* illnesses may also cause exterior pathogens to move inward, *chái hú* (bupleurum [root]) and *huáng qín* (scutellaria [root]) on the one hand meet and confront the pathogen. On the other hand, this confrontation produces a cease fire but no reconciliation. This is because the pathogen and the correct qi cannot exist together side by side. It is not that the correct is victorious over the pathogen, rather the pathogen is victorious over the correct; these two cannot be essentially regulated and harmonized. The intent of the treatment methods of harmonization and resolution is to harmonize the interior and resolve the exterior. For in harmonizing the interior the pathogen is not allowed to attack, and in resolving the exterior the pathogen is allowed to exteriorize. While the intent remains focused on dispelling the pathogen, the tactics employed must vary with variations in the pathocondition. It can be deduced from these prescription methods that whenever strong calming of the interior with simultaneous resistance to foreign aggression is employed, this approach falls within the category of harmonization and resolution. [A prescription representative of this approach is:]

Huò Xiāng Zhèng Qì Sǎn (Agastache/Patchouli Qi-Righting Powder)
from *Hé Jì Jú Fāng*

tǔ huò xiāng	agastache
zǐ sū yè	perilla leaf
bái zhǐ	angelica dahurica
fú líng	poria
bái zhú	ovate atractylodes [root]
chén pí	tangerine peel
bàn xià	pinellia [tuber]
dà fù pí	areca husk
hòu pò	magnolia bark
jié gěng	platycodon [root]
gān cǎo	licorice [root]
jiāng	ginger
dà zǎo	jujube [fruit]

This treats external contraction of wind cold, internal injury due to dampness, and food [accumulation] with symptoms [such as] chills and fever, headache, nausea, and thoraco-diaphragmatic fullness and oppression. *Tǔ huò xiāng* (agastache) is the sovereign medicinal that courses, dissipates, and harmonizes the middle, simultaneously treating the exterior and the interior. *Zǐ sū yè* (perilla leaf), *bái zhǐ* (angelica dahurica) and *jié gěng* (platycodon [root]) dissipate cold and disinhibit the diaphragm, as well as assist promoting the exterior [i.e.: diaphoresis]. *Hòu pò* (magnolia bark), *dà fù pí* (areca husk), *chén pí* (tangerine peel), and *bàn xià* (pinellia [tuber]), transform dampness, digest food [i.e.: enhance digestion] and circulate the qi, as well as assist coursing the interior. *Fú líng* (poria), *bái zhú* (ovate atractylodes [root]), and *gān cǎo* (licorice [root]) are used to supplement and disinhibit the correct qi.[5]

---

[5]Trans: the idea here is not to harmonize the correct qi and the pathogen. These are totally incompatible. What is being harmonized is the environment of the interior itself. The pathogen is resolved to the exterior.

7. METHODS FOR ABATING FEVER BY JOINT RESOLUTION OF THE EXTERIOR AND THE INTERIOR

Diaphoresis is appropriate for exterior heat, and interior heat should be cleared by precipitation. These are the major methods indicated in these cases. If, at an early stage of illness, exterior and interior symptoms are seen together or, if exterior symptoms are not resolved after many days and interior symptoms also appear, one may then work along two lines. [These two approaches are:] coursing the exterior and clearing the interior, and these are together referred to as methods for resolving both the exterior and the interior. [A prescription representative of this method is:]

Sān Huáng Shí Gāo Tāng (Three Yellows and Gypsum Decoction)	
from *Táo Jié ān Fāng*	
shí gāo	gypsum
huáng qín	scutellaria [root]
huáng lián	coptis [root]
huáng bǎi	phellodendron [bark]
shān zhī zǐ	gardenia [fruit]
má huáng	ephedra
dòu chǐ	fermented soybean
jiāng	ginger
dà zǎo	jujube [fruit]

This treats both the exterior and the interior as well as heat above and below with a flooding rapid pulse. One simply cannot use *Má Huáng Tāng* (Ephedra Decoction) or *Bái Hǔ Tāng* (White Tiger Decoction). However, both these prescriptions are based on *má huáng* (ephedra) and *dòu chǐ* (fermented soybean), which resolve exterior heat. *Shí gāo* (gypsum), *shān zhī zǐ* (gardenia [fruit]), *huáng lián* (coptis [root]), and *huáng qín* (scutellaria [root]) resolve heat in all three burners. [One should use] the [following] complex prescription:

Fáng Fēng Tōng Shèng Sǎn (Ledebouriella Sage-Inspired Powder)	
from *Liú Hé Jiān Fāng*	
fáng fēng	ledebouriella [root]
jīng jiè suì	schizonepeta spike
lián qiáo	forsythia [fruit]
má huáng	ephedra
bò hé	mint
chuān xiōng	ligusticum [root]
dāng guī	tangkuei
bái sháo yào	white peony [root]
bái zhú	ovate atractylodes [root]
shān zhī zǐ	gardenia [fruit]
dà huáng	rhubarb
máng xiāo	mirabilite
huáng qín	scutellaria [root]
huá shí	talcum
shí gāo	gypsum
jié gěng	platycodon [root]
gān cǎo	licorice [root]
xiè bái	Chinese chive [bulb]
jiāng	ginger

[This prescription] treats aversion to chill, high fever, reddening of the eyes, nasal obstruction, bitter taste and dryness in the mouth, cough, difficulty in swallowing and breathing, constipation, and darkened reddened urine. *Má huáng* (ephedra), *fáng fēng* (ledebouriella [root]), *jīng jiè suì* (schizonepeta spike), *bò hé* (mint), and *jié gěng* (platycodon [root]) are used to diffuse the lung and dissipate wind; *lián qiáo* (forsythia [fruit]), *fú líng* (poria), *shí gāo* (gypsum), and *huá shí* (talcum) clear heat from the interior. *Máng xiāo* (mirabilite) and *dà huáng* (rhubarb) drain repletion and free the stools. Also, because the appetite is affected and the qi and blood are depressed, *dāng guī* (tangkuei), *bái sháo yào* (white peony [root]), *chuān xiōng* (ligusticum [root]), *bái zhú* (ovate atractylodes [root]), and *gān cǎo* (licorice [root]) are incorporated to regulate the liver and strengthen the spleen.

Analyzed in this way, the logic is clear. The complex symptom patterns indicated above in the use of prescription methods for abating fever are nonetheless clear and definite and should be considered from a variety of viewpoints. The foundational theories of Chinese medicine determine the manner in which Chinese medical compounds are organized.

In Chinese medicine, exterior patterns are divided into three phases, the earliest being the *tài yáng* channel, the next being the *yáng míng* channel, followed by the *shào yáng* channel. Together they are referred to as the "three yang channels" and the invasion of all these is characterized by fever.

[To summmarize] the symptoms differentiated in the above narration: for *tài yáng* with aversion to cold and fever, *má huáng* (ephedra) is the main medicinal used; for *yáng míng* with no aversion to cold but with fever, *gé gēn* (pueraria [root]) is the main medicinal used; and for the *shào yáng* with alternating chills and fever, *chái hú* (bupleurum [root]) is the main medicinal used. Nevertheless, as an external pathogen progresses, two channels may also be seen to be [simultaneously] affected and they must be dealt with together. For instance, for a combined *tài yáng–yáng míng* illness, [the following prescription] is indicated:

Gé Gēn Tāng (Pueraria Decoction)	
Zhāng Zhòngjǐng's prescription	
gé gēn	pueraria [root]
má huáng	ephedra
guì zhī	cinnamon twig
bái sháo yào	white peony [root]
gān ǎo	licorice [root]
jiāng	ginger
dà zǎo	jujube [fruit]

For a combined *yáng míng–shào yáng* illness, use of [the following prescription] is indicated:

Chái Hú Shēng Má Tāng (Bupleurum and Cimicifuga Decoction)	
from *Hé Jì Jú Fāng*	
chái hú	bupleurum [root]
gé gēn	pueraria [root]
qián hú	peucedanum [root]
huáng qín	scutellaria [root]
shēng má	cimicifuga [root]
sāng bái pí	mulberry root bark
jīng jiè suì	schizonepeta spike
chì sháo yào	red peony [root]
shí gāo	gypsum
dòu chǐ	fermented soybean
jiāng	ginger

By the same token there may be interior symptoms of a simultaneous illness of the upper and middle burners, simultaneous illnesses of the middle and lower burner, or simultaneous illnesses of all the burners as well, and these also must be addressed simultaneously. All these strategies are referred to as methods for dual resolution.

8. Methods for Clearing and Transforming Damp-heat

Dampness is a yin pathogen, and heat is a yang pathogen. While they differ as to their essential nature, they may be combined like oil in wheat flour, resulting in a [condition] that is not easily dissipated. Damp febrile illnesses most obviously present themselves [in a manner reminiscent of] the peeling away [of an onion skin], removing one layer and exposing another in a never-ending manner. The characteristics of damp warm illnesses are generalized heat symptoms such as fever that increases in the afternoon, chilled feet, dry mouth with no thirst, preference for warm soups, headache, spontaneous sweating, and cardiac vexation. There are also damp symptoms such as thoracic oppression, nausea, and a thick slimy tongue moss. If the condition is serious, there will be spirit clouding, wherein the patient may be sometimes lucid and sometimes confused in a manner similar to that of sleep but which is not actually sleep. This is distinct from the heat symptoms of insomnia that is due to manic vexation, as the etiology is due to the enshroudment of damp-heat which hoodwinks the clear yang, and is thus not the same condition as a heat pathogen invading the brain and causing the spirit to lose its normal function.

Therapeutic prescription methods are primarily those of clearing heat and transforming dampness. Nonetheless, if the damp heat tends to predominate, it is important to consider the relative importance of the various medicinals used, as there should be simultaneous combination of prescription methods for diffusing and outthrusting, soothing depression, and bland percolation, as well as medicinals that are aromatic, bitter, and dry to break the force of the illness. The following are examples of typically-used formulas:

Sān Rén Tāng (Three Kernels Decoction)	
Wú Jútōng's prescription	
xìng rén	apricot kernel
yì yǐ rén	coix [seed]
huá shí	talcum
tōng cǎo	rice-paper plant pith
zhú yè	black bamboo leaf
hòu pò	magnolia bark
bàn xià	pinellia [tuber]
bái dòu kòu	cardamom

The *zhú yè* (black bamboo leaf) and *huá shí* (talcum) are clearing; the *hòu pò* (magnolia bark), *bàn xià* (pinellia [tuber]) and *bái dòu kòu* (cardamom) are drying; the *xìng rén* (apricot kernel) is diffusing; the *tōng cǎo* (rice-paper plant pith) and the *yì yǐ rén* (coix [seed]) are disinhibiting. [Another example is:]

Gān Lù Xiāo Dú Dān (Sweet Dew Toxin-Dispersing Elixir)	
Yè Tiānshì's prescription	
tǔ huò xiāng	agastache
bái dòu kòu	cardamom
shí chāng pú	acorus [root]
wū shàn	belamcanda [root]
bò hé	mint
yīn chén hāo	capillaris
huá shí	talcum
bèi mǔ	fritillaria [bulb]
huáng qín	scutellaria [root]
lián qiáo	forsythia [fruit]
mù tōng	mutong [stem]

Huáng qín (scutellaria [root]) and *huá shí* (talcum) are cooling. *Bái dòu kòu* (cardamom) is acrid. *Bò hé* (mint) is light and spreads. *Tǔ huò xiāng* (agastache) is aromatic. *Shí chāng pú* (acorus [root]) opens the orifices. *Bèi mǔ* (fritillaria [bulb]) transforms phlegm. *Wū shàn* (belamcanda [root]) benefits the throat. *Mù tōng* (mutong [stem]) guides the urine, and the addition of *lián qiáo* (forsythia [fruit]) and *yīn chén hāo* (capillaris) is good for clearing and transforming damp-heat in the lower burner. Thus, the prescription is organized in a most meticulous manner.

[The following prescription] is most often chosen for the treatment of spirit clouding due to damp-heat:

Shén Xī Dán (Spirit-Like Rhinoceros Horn Elixir)	
from *Wēn Rè Jīng Wěi Fāng*	
xiān dì huáng	fresh rehmannia [root]
zǐ cǎo	puccoon
bǎn lán gēn	isatis root
dòu chǐ	fermented soybean
tiān huā fěn	trichosanthes root
lián qiáo	forsythia fruit
xuán shēn	scrophularia [root]
rén zhōng huáng	licorce in human feces
huáng qín	scutellaria [root]
xī jiǎo	rhinoceros horn
jīn yín huā	lonicera [flower]
shí chāng pú	acorus [root]

It clears heat and settles the middle [burner] while simultaneously transforming turbidity and opening the orifices, thus addressing both etiologies in the illness.

In jaundice patterns with fever there will be perspiration from the head but no bodily perspiration, urinary inhibition, thirst, thoracic oppression, nausea, and skin which is bright [yellow] like the color of *jú zǐ* (citrus seeds). This is referred to as infectious hepatitis in Western medicine and is classified as a yang jaundice pattern in Chinese medicine. [The following prescription] is used to clear and disinhibit:

Yīn Chén Hào Tāng (Capillaris Decoction)	
Zhāng Zhòngjǐng's prescription	
yīn chén hāo	capillaris
shān zhī zǐ	gardenia [fruit]
dà huáng	rhubarb

It is my experience that infectious hepatitis is a type of jaundice, and while the jaundice may not yet have developed, the jaundice will be preceded by the appearance of dark yellow urine. Therefore, in Chinese medicine, the ideal prescription methods are those for clearing, transforming, and disinhibiting the urine, so as to actually prevent the development of the jaundice and thus the infectious hepatitis.

9. Methods for Abating Fever by Clearing the Constructive and Resolving Toxins

In febrile patterns, aside from discriminating exterior and interior, then discriminating between patterns related to the three yang and the triple burner within the context of exterior and interior, it is important to discriminate the defensive, qi, constructive, and blood aspects. If a pathogen has already invaded the constructive and blood aspects, simply treating the protective and the qi aspects is inappropriate. Nevertheless, we cannot hurriedly employ methods for cooling the blood and checking reckless blood flow. For instance, if a warm pathogen causes the development of macules, then the use of [the following] prescription is indicated because the formula includes sweet and cold medicinals that clear the stomach:

Huà Bān Tāng (Macule-Transforming Decoction)	
Wú Jútōng's prescription	
xī jiǎo	rhinoceros horn
xuán shēn	scrophularia [root]
zhī mǔ	anemarrhena [root]
shí gāo	gypsum
gān cǎo	licorice [root]
gǔ yá	rice sprout

For pediatric measles, the use of [the following prescription] is indicated:

Zhú Yè Liù Bàng Tāng (Bamboo Leaf, Tamarisk and Arctium Decoction)	
Miào Zhòngchún's prescription	
xī hé liǔ	tamarisk [twig and leaf]
jīng jiè suì	schizonepeta spike
bò hé	mint
gān cǎo	licorice [root]
gé gēn	pueraria [root]
niú bàng zǐ	arctium [seed]
zhú ye	black bamboo leaf
shí gāo	gypsum
xuán shēn	scrophularia [root]
mài mén dōng	ophiopogon [tuber]
chuán tuì	cicada molting

[This is] because medicinals for clearing and draining blood heat must be included in formulas that are acrid, cooling, and exterior-resolving. If there is a dramatic development of macules and papules, the first treatment method indicated is the promotion of their eruption. This development means that the pathogen has clearly entered the constructive aspect. Therefore, the addition of medicinals for cooling the blood aspect is indicated. At this point the relative depths of the constructive and blood aspects have been distinguished. When a pathogen enters the constructive aspect, changes may still be expected in the qi aspect [that is, changes that require treatment in addition to treatment of the constructive aspect], yet when it lies in the blood, the blood must be directly cleared and cooled.

When a pathogen enters the constructive/blood aspects, and the symptoms are extremely severe, and include spiritual stupor, agitative mania, and fright reversal, which Chinese medicine understands as heat entering the pericardium, one may use [one of the following prescriptions]:

Zǐ Xuě Dān (Purple Snow Elixir)	
from *Běn Shì Fāng*	
cí shí	loadstone
shí gāo	gypsum
fāng jiě shí	calcite
huá shí	talcum
líng yáng jiǎo	antelope horn
mù xiāng	saussurea [root]
xī jiǎo	rhinoceros horn
chén xiāng	aquilaria [wood]
dīng xiāng	clove
shēng má	cimicifuga [root]
xuán shēn	scrophularia [root]
gān cǎo	licorice [root]

Niú Huáng Qīng Xīn Wán (Bovine Bezoar Heart-Clearing Pill)	
from *Wàn Sì Fàng*'s prescription	
niú huáng	bovine bezoar
huáng lián	coptis
huáng qín	scutellaria [root]
yù jīn	curcuma [tuber]
zhū shā	cinnabar
shān zhī zǐ	gardenia [fruit]

I believe that this is indicative of a viral infection of the brain and central nervous system causing confusion, therefore, it indicates the use of medicinals which tend to be settling as well as heat-clearing and toxin-resolving.

When pathogenic heat enters the constructive aspect, this easily causes symptoms of epistaxis and blood mixed with phlegm. Whenever there are febrile symptoms, methods for clearing the constructive aspect and cooling the blood aspect are most often used, and hemostatic methods are not called for. This is because there is frenetic movement of the blood due to its being heated. If the constructive aspect is not cleared, then the bleeding will not be arrested. As an example of treatment we can use a modification of [the following]:

Yù Nǔ Jiān (Jade Lady Brew)
Wú Jútōng's prescription

xiān dì huáng	raw fresh rehmannia [root]
zhī mǔ	anemarrhena [root]
shí gāo	gypsum
xuán shēn	scrophularia [root]
mài mén dōng	ophiopogon [tuber]

It treats blazing of both the qi and the blood. If the condition is grave, the use of [the following prescription will] abate the fever and arrest bleeding:

Xī Jiǎo Dì Huáng Tāng (Rhinoceros Horn and Rehmannia Decoction)
from Jì Shēng Fāng's prescription

xī jiǎo	rhinoceros horn
xiān dì huáng	raw fresh rehmannia [root]
chì sháo yào	red peony [root]
mǔ dān pí	moutan [root bark]

10. METHODS FOR ABATING FEVER BY SOOTHING DEPRESSION

The five viscera may all exhibit depressive symptoms and, where there is depression, fever may develop. The seven emotions provide the predominant etiology of the above[-mentioned] depressions, and the liver and gallbladder channels are most often affected of all the viscera and bowels. The symptom pattern includes afternoon fever or alternating chills and fever, or a sensation of a sudden upsurge of heat when irritable; an abundance of blood in the face, agitated emotional state, becoming easily irritated and annoyed, a sensation of pressure in the head, tinnitus, insomnia where one is often frightened awake, and irregular menses in women. Depressive liver patterns will quite easily influence the stomach and spleen, and often will be accompanied by symptoms of anorexia, thoracic oppression, eructation, and constipation. In treatment, it is appropriate to course and free the liver qi, for if the liver qi possesses its quality of orderly reaching, then the fire will dissipate of its own accord, the blood will harmonize itself, and digestion will naturally return to normalcy. [The formula of choice is]:

Xiāo Yáo Sǎn (Free Wanderer Powder)
from *Hé Jì Jú Fāng*

chái hú	bupleurum [root]
dāng guī	tangkuei
bái sháo yào	white peony [root]
bò hé	mint
bái zhú	ovate atractylodes [root]
fú líng	poria
gān cǎo	licorice [root]
pào jiāng	blast-fried ginger

This is a commonly used formula which primarily regulates the liver qi and diffuses and frees the yang qi. Assisting these functions, it harmonizes and nourishes the spleen and stomach to resolve depression. [The following formula] strongly rectifies the qi, clears fire, and has a similar use.

Huà Gān Jiān (Liver-Transforming Brew)
from *Wèi Yù Huáng Fāng*

qīng pí	unripe tangerine peel
chén pí	tangerine peel
bái sháo yào	white peony [root]
bèi mǔ	fritillaria [bulb]
shān zhī zǐ	gardenia [fruit]
zé xiè	alisma [tuber]

Chronic depressive symptoms may cause a desiccation of blood fluids, emaciation of the flesh, bone steaming and taxation depression, as well as cervical scrofula and amenorrhea. While this is similar to vacuity taxation and, for that matter, may become vacuity taxation, it is nonetheless inappropriate to rely solely on supplementing prescriptions, as bitter, acrid, cooling and moistening, diffusing and freeing methods are indicated. Bitter is able to drain heat, acrid is able to rectify the qi, cool and moistening medicinals enrich dryness, diffusing and freeing medicinals dissipate depression. When treating emotional illnesses, the property of the medicinals used must comply with the nature of the condition. This is because therapy will be effective only when softness conquers rigidity. This is reflected in the composition of prescriptions such as modified *Xiāo Yán Sǎn* (Free Wanderer Powder), and *Huà Gān Jiān* or in *Zuǒ Jīn Wǎn* (Left-Running Metal Pill), Zhū Dānxī's prescription containing *huáng lián* (coptis [root]) and *wú zhū yú* (evodia [fruit]).

11. METHODS FOR ABATING FEVER BY DISPELLING STASIS

Fever with manic symptoms differs from heat entering the pericardium in that there is a simultaneous urgent binding in the lower abdomen *[xiào fù]*, and normal urination. This falls into to the category of blood accumulation and [the following prescription] is indicated:

Táo Rén Chéng Qì Tāng (Peach Kernel Qi-Infusing Decoction)
Zhāng Zhòngjǐng's prescription

táo rén	peach kernel
guì zhī	cinnamon twig
dà huáng	rhubarb
máng xiāo	mirabilite
gān cǎo	licorice [root]

Also, if there are *shào yáng* channel symptoms such as alternating fever and chills or delirious speech immediately preceding or proceeding from menstruation, and binding pain in the costal and umbilical regions, this is from heat entering the blood chamber. Measures for clearing heat and dispelling stasis are also used in prescriptions such as:

Táo Sì Xiào Chǎi Hú Tāng (Master Tao's Minor Bupleurum Decoction)	
Tao Jiēān's prescription	
chái hú	bupleurum [root]
huáng qín	scutellaria [root]
bàn xià	pinellia [tuber]
xiān dì huáng	raw fresh rehmannia [root]
mǔ dān pí	moutan [root bark]
táo rén	peach kernel
shān zhā	crataegus [fruit]
gān cǎo	licorice [root]

This prescription is indicated for intestinal welling-abscess, which is similar to acute appendicitis and characterized by low abdominal pain that intensifies with pressure, and inability to turn on the side, relatively smooth thigh flexion and generalized fever. In the early stages, urgent removal of stasis is also indicated, with administration of [the following prescription] to attack it:

Dà Huáng Mǒu Dān Pí Tāng (Rhubarb and Moutan Decoction)	
Zhāng Zhòngjǐng's prescription	
dà huáng	rhubarb
mǔ dān pí	moutan [root bark]
táo rén	peach kernel
dōng guā zǐ	wax gourd seed
máng xiāo	mirabilite

For fever due to external swelling sores, since it is most often due to the onset of qi stasis and congelation, Chinese medicine values the internal administration of medicines used to abate heat and dissipate [the pathogen]. This is none other than harmonizing the constructive and quickening the blood, and there are numerous examples of this practice.

It is my belief that the utilization of "qi" within the human body is unique to the medicine of our homeland, and from the qi there is a mutual generation of "blood." Qi and blood are considered to be extremely important in Chinese medicine; qi depression and blood stasis are given much attention in pathology. This is because in their impairment of physiological functions they can engender a great variety of illnesses. Fever is a generalized symptom and the therapeutic methods used must be global. We must have a deep understanding of both depressive and stasis symptoms.

12. METHODS FOR ABATING FEVER BY ABDUCTION AND DISPERSAL

Abating fever by methods of abduction and dispersal is frequently used for gastrointestinal illnesses that are caused by afflictions such as dietary intemperance or food poisoning which cause symptoms such as those associated with gastritis and enteritis. For such commonly seen symptoms as digestate accumulation, stomach pain due to overeating, nausea and vomiting, eructation of sour fluid, or abdominal pain and diarrhea with an intermittent generalized fever that suddenly becomes elevated, one may use [the following prescription]:

Băo Hé Wán (Harmony-Preserving Pill)	
Zhū Dānxī's prescription	
shén qū	medicated leaven
shān zhā	crataegus [fruit]
lái fú zǐ	radish seed
bàn xià	pinellia [tuber]
chén pí	tangerine peel
mài yá	barley sprout
fú líng	poria
lián qiáo	forsythia [fruit]

If the food stasis is digested, then the fever will abate on its own. Furthermore, acute dysentery with abdominal pain and generalized fever is most often due to accumulation and stasis in the intestines. Use [the following prescription] to remove the accumulation:

Zhǐ Shí Dǎo Zhì Wán (Unripe Bitter Orange Stagnation-Abducting Pill)	
Lǐ Dōngyuán's prescription	
dà huáng	rhubarb
zhǐ shí	unripe bitter orange
huáng qín	scutellaria [root]
huáng lián	coptis [root]
shén qū	medicated leaven
bái zhú	ovate atractylodes [root]
fú líng	poria
zé xiè	alisma [tuber]

The heat will follow suit and be resolved as well.

Fever in the early stages of dysentery is not considered to be a serious condition in Chinese medicine. However, in the case of unchecked long-standing diarrhea and dysentery, if there is basically no heat involved and then a fever develops, this fever is not due to the development of the condition related to the contraction of an external pathogen. Thus, it is extremely important [to attend to this development because] it is most often due to an injury of the yin and therefore dispersive abducting and coursing dispersive methods are contraindicated. This situation requires the use of prescriptions such as:

Ē Jiāo Liáng Méi Wán (Ass Hide Glue, Coptis, and Mume Decoction)	
from Zhèng Zhì Zhǔn Shéng	
lù jiǎo jiāo	deerhorn glue
huáng lián	coptis [root]
wū méi	mume
dāng guī	tangkuei
chì sháo yào	red peony [root]
fú líng	poria
huáng bǎi	phellodendron [bark]
pào jiāng	blast-fried ginger

Pediatric gan accumulation with tidal fever in the skin and muscle, emaciation which progresses daily, lusterless complexion, and umbilical distension and vexation agitation with copious crying is also due to an unrestrained diet injuring the form of the stomach and intestines. Dispersing abducting and middle harmonizing methods may be used in the early stages, but after it develops further, methods for supplementing the middle, clearing heat, and digesting and grinding accumulation are also used in simultaneous consideration of the root and branch in prescriptions such as:

Féi Ér Wán (Chubby Child Pill)	
from *Yī Zōng Jīn Jiàn Fāng*	
rén shēn	ginseng
bái zhú	ovate atractylodes [root]
huáng lián	coptis [root]
fú líng	poria
shǐ jūn zǐ	quisqualis [fruit]
shén qū	medicated leaven
mài yá	barley sprout
shān zhā	crataegus [fruit]
gān cǎo	licorice [root]
lú huì	aloe

13. METHODS FOR ABATING FEVER BY COMBATING MALARIA

[In times past], Chinese medicine had for the most part no idea of what causes malaria. Nevertheless, from very early on our ancestors recorded prescriptions that were primarily for [treating] malaria, such as [the following prescriptions]:

Chán Shān Yǐn (Dichroa Beverage)	
from *Hé Jì Jú Fāng*	
cháng shān	dichroa [root]
cǎo guǒ	tsaoko [fruit]
bīn láng	areca [nut]
zhī mǔ	anemarrhena [root]
wū méi	mume [fruit]
jiāng	ginger
bèi mǔ	fritillaria [bulb]

Qī Bǎo Yǐn (Seven Jewel Beverage)	
from *Yì Jiǎn Fāng*	
cháng shān	dichroa [root]
bái dòu kòu	cardamom
bīn láng	areca [nut]
qīng pí	unripe tangerine peel
hòu pò	magnolia bark
chén pí	tangerine peel
gān cǎo	licorice [root]

Both prescriptions employ *cháng shān* (dichroa [root]) to combat
malaria. Based on modern research, the capacity of dichroa to combat
malaria far exceeds that of quinine. This is another example of the exquisite substances contained in the medicine of our homeland.

[Those suffering from] acute malaria will exhibit initial chills followed
by fever, one episode per day, every other, or every third day, and the diagnosis is comparatively clear. Nonetheless, the types of fever [each patient
may present with] are not always identical. The chills may precede the
fever, the fever may precede the chills; the chills may be severe and the
fever slight; there may be fever and no chills; it may develop in the morning, in the afternoon or during the night. Since the same illness may have
differing symptoms, Chinese medicine distinguishes between phlegm
malaria, cold malaria, bi malaria, and three yin malaria. Formulations
such as [the following] have all been settled upon [as useful prescriptions
for malaria]:

Chái Pò Tāng (Bupleurum and Magnolia Bark Decoction)	
from *Zhèng Zhì Zhǔn Shéng*	
chái hú	bupleurum [root]
hòu pò	magnolia bark
dú huó	tuhuo [angelica root]
qián hú	peucedanum [root]
huáng qín	scutellaria [root]
cāng zhú	atractylodes [root]
chén pí	tangerine peel
bàn xià	pinellia [tuber]
fú líng	poria
tǔ huò xiāng	agastache
gān cǎo	licorice [root]

Shǔ Qī Sǎn (Qi-Smoothing Powder)	
Zhāng Zhòngjǐng's prescription	
shǔ qī	dichroa leaf
yún mǔ fán	alum
lóng gǔ	dragon bone

Guì Zhī Huáng Tāng (Cinnamon Twig and Scutellaria Decoction)	
from *Zhèng Zhì Zhǔn Shéng*	
guì zhī	cinnamon twig
huáng qín	scutellaria [root]
rén shēn	ginseng
gān cǎo	licorice [root]
chái hú	bupleurum [root]
bàn xià	pinellia [tuber]
shí gāo	gypsum
zhī mǔ	anemarrhena [root]

Chái Hú Xióng Guī Tāng (Bupleurum, Ligusticum, and Tangkuei Decoction)	
from Shěn Sǐ Zhūn Shēng Shū	
chái hú	bupleurum [root]
chuān xiōng	ligusticum [root]
dāng guī	tangkuei
jié gěng	platycodon [root]
chì sháo yào	red peony [root]
rén shēn	ginseng
hòu pò	magnolia bark
bái zhú	ovate atractylodes [root]
fú líng	poria
qīng pí	unripe tangerine peel
gé gēn	pueraria [root]
hóng huā	carthamus [flower]
gān cǎo	licorice [root]
wū méi	mume [fruit]
jiāng	ginger
dà zǎo	jujube [fruit]

Here, therapy is based on the symptom pattern, and cháng shān (dichroa [root]) is not used as a medicinal of special effect.

Malaria may easily destroy the red blood cells, creating hepatic impoverishment in which there is not only a lusterless complexion and a weakness of the extremities, but also, [a condition where] the patient's motivation does not recover as the chills and fever cease, and the chills and fever return upon exertion. This is referred to as taxation malaria, and is treated by supplementing and nourishing the qi and blood, using prescriptions such as:

Mr. He's Beverage	
Zhāng Jǐngyuè's prescription	
hé shǒu wū	flowery knotweed [root]
rén shēn	ginseng
dāng guī	tangkuei
chén pí	tangerine peel
pài jiāng	blast-fried ginger
dà zǎo	jujube [fruit]

Longstanding malaria with splenomegaly presenting with a left subcostal hardness and fullness that is like concretions and conglomerations, and chills and fever that follow exertion, is referred to as malarial lump glomus. In these cases [the following prescription] is employed to harmonize the blood and dissipate stasis:

Mother of Malaria Pills	
from Zhèng Zhì Zhǔn Shéng Fāng	
biē jiǎ	turtle shell
qīng pí	unripe tangerine peel
é zhú	zedoary
sān léng	sparganium [root]
táo rén	peach kernel
shén qū	medicated leaven
hǎi fěn	notarchus filament
xiāng fù zǐ	cyperus [root]
hóng huā	carthamus [flower]
mài yá	barley sprout

This provides an explanation of the symptomatic treatment of malaria in Chinese medicine, while simultaneously taking the discrimination of syndromes into consideration in carrying out treatment.

14. METHODS FOR ABATING FEVER BY AVERTING EPIDEMIC

Epidemic patterns are indicative of an infectious pathogen characterized by foul turbidity. This type of pathogen will most frequently attack
the intestines and stomach directly, having been contracted by respiration
through the mouth and nose, resulting in initial symptoms of cephalic
dizziness and brain distension, a slight aversion to cold in the spine, nausea and thoracic oppression, or diarrhea with periumbilical pain and high
fever that is unresolved even after diaphoresis. Moreover, it is often the
case that upon administration of medicines there is diaphoresis and the
fever is diminished, but is not completely resolved. Typically, the fever
will appear to be deep-lying or the fever will abate but, after two or three
days, it will return. It can be seen that the accumulation of the internal
pathogen has not been transmitted from the interior to the exterior and
that the remaining pathogen must be thoroughly dissipated. In general,
[the following prescription] is used with the intent of outthrusting and
draining the pathogen from the interior:

Dá Yuán Yǐn (**Membrane-Source-Opening Beverage**)	
Wú Yòukè's prescription	
huáng qín	scutellaria [root]
bái sháo yào	white peony [root]
hòu pò	magnolia bark
cǎo guǒ	tsaoko [fruit]
zhī mǔ	anemarrhena [root]
bīn láng	areca [nut]
gān cǎo	licorice [root]
jiāng	ginger
dà zǎo	jujube [fruit]

In the case of massive head scourge[6] and thermic epidemic symptoms,
there will be fever at the onset, dry mouth and tongue, sore throat, gradual reddening of the head and face, and an inability to open the eyes.
[Use] prepared prescriptions such as:

Pǔ Jì Xiāo Dú Yǐn (**Universal Salvation Toxin-Dispersing Beverage**)	
Lǐ Dōngyuán's prescription	
huáng qín	scutellaria [root]
huáng lián	coptis [root]
jú hóng	red tangerine peel
gān cǎo	licorice [root]
xuán shēn	scrophularia [root]
lián qiáo	forsythia [fruit]
bǎn lán gēn	isatis root
mǎ bó	puffball
niú bàng zǐ	arctium [seed]
bò hé	mint
bái jiāng cán	silkworm
shēng má	cimicifuga [root]
chái hú	bupleurum [root]
jié gěng	platycodon [root]

---

[6]*Dà tóu wēn*: A disease that results from the invasion of the spleen and stomach channels by
seasonal wind-warmth toxin and that is characterized by swelling and redness of the head,
and sometimes by painful swelling of the throat, and, in severe cases, signs such as deafness,
clenched jaw, clouded spirit, and delirious raving.

[This prescription] uses the acrid, cool *bò hé* (mint), *niú bàng zǐ* (arctium [seed]), and *lián qiáo* (forsythia [fruit]) to dissipate wind heat. [It] uses the bitter cold *huáng qín* (scutellaria [root]) and *huáng lián* (coptis [root]) to drain repletion fire, course the qi with *chái hú* (bupleurum [root]), *shēng má* (cimicifuga [root]), *jié gěng* (platycodon [root]), and *jú hóng* (red tangerine peel), and dissipate swelling with *bái jiāng cán* (silkworm), *mǎ bó* (puffball), and *gān cǎo* (licorice [root]). Because this illness is related to the blood aspect, *xuán shēn* (scrophularia [root]) and *bǎn lán gēn* (isatis root) are also used to move the blood and resolve toxins. There are a great number of epidemic symptoms and of these only two types are represented here to demonstrate the variety of therapeutic approaches.

15. METHODS FOR ABATING FEVER BY WARMING THE CHANNELS

External contraction with fever at the onset, fatigue, and lassitude and a sinking rather than floating pulse, is due to a weakened body and an extreme vacuity of yang. Although this is a contraction of wind-cold, diaphoresis is not indicated because diaphoresis may easily result in the collapse of yang and thus vacuity desertion. However, one must eliminate the pathogen, because its force exploits the vacuity and [it will then] directly penetrate to a greater depth if it is not dissipated. This is a joint *tài yáng* and *shào yīn* illness; treatment is aimed primarily at warming the channels. Warming the channels implies warming the *shào yīn* channels to promote the defensive functions. These methods are assisted by dispersing medicinals which eliminate the exterior pathogen from the *tài yáng*. This condition calls for the use of prescriptions such as:

Má Huáng Fù Zǐ Xì Xīn Tāng (Ephedra, Aconite, and Asarum Decoction)	
Zhāng Zhòngjǐng's prescription	
má huáng	ephedra
fù zǐ	aconite accessory tuber
xì xīn	asarum

The *fù zǐ* (aconite accessory tuber) warms the *shào yīn* and assists the yang qi; *má huáng* (ephedra) dissipates wind cold from the *tài yáng,* and *xì xīn* (asarum) is an exterior medicinal used for the *shào yìn* and as a liason between the exterior and the interior. The simplicity of the medicinal tastes included in this formula strongly demonstrate its therapeutic focus.

These symptoms are quite uncommon and the treatment methods are similar to those of harmonization and resolution, as well as joint resolution of the interior and exterior, although in actuality they differ in some regards. This condition also differs from fever due to external contraction in a weakened patient. In general, a weakened constitution is more susceptible to external contractions and, as a result, there are chills and fever and spontaneous perspiration that is most often a consequence of an insecurity of the defensive qi. [In this case the following prescription] is used to secure the exterior and eliminate the pathogen:

Yù Píng Fēng Sǎn (Jade Wind-Barrier Powder)	
from *Sì Yǐ Dé Xiào*	
huáng qí	astragalus [root]
fáng fēng	ledebouriella [root]
bái zhú	ovate atractylodes [root]

16. METHODS FOR ABATING FEVER BY ENRICHING THE YIN

Chinese medicine divides illness into the two major categories of external contraction and internal injury. Measures for enriching the yin and abating fever are used for vacuity symptoms due to internal injury. Vacuity patterns, where the fever is more often than not mild, can be further divided into three categories. One is yin vacuity; this is characterized by bodily emaciation, fever in the five hearts, elevation of body temperature in the afternoon, and awareness of a steaming sensation between the bones and flesh. [Yin vacuity is treated with] prescriptions such as:

Qīng Gǔ Sǎn (Bone-Clearing Powder)	
from *Zhèng Zhì Zhǔn Shéng*	
yín chái hú	lanceolate stellaria [root]
huáng lián	coptis [root]
dì gǔ pí	lycium root bark
qīng hāo yè	sweet wormwood leaf
zhī mǔ	anemarrhena [root]
biē jiǎ	turtle shell
qín jiāo	large gentian [root]
gān cǎo	licorice [root]

These fevers are all a result of injury to the yin aspect. If the yin is injured, then there will be an effulgence of liver and gallbladder fire, so *biē jiǎ* (turtle shell) is used to nourish the yin; *dì gǔ pí* (lycium root bark), *huáng lián* (coptis [root]), and *zhī mǔ* (anemarrhena [root]) eliminate heat from the yin aspect and balance it internally. The *yín chái hú* (lanceolate stellaria [root]) and *qīng hāo* (sweet wormwood) eliminate fire from the liver and gallbladder and dissipate the exterior. These are the general methods for abating vacuity heat.

Cases of pulmonary consumption characterized by cough, bodily weakness, and spontaneous perspiration are treated by prescriptions such as:

Qín Jiāo Fú Léi Tāng (Large Gentian Emaciation Decoction)	
from *Zhǐ Zhǐ Fāng*	
chái hú	bupleurum [root]
qín jiāo	large gentian [root]
biē jiǎ	turtle shell
rén shēn	ginseng
dāng guī	tangkuei
dì gǔ pí	lycium root bark
zǐ wǎn	aster [root]
bàn xià	pinellia [tuber]
gān cǎo	licorice [root]
jiāng	ginger
dà zǎo	jujube [fruit]

Also, for the treatment of wind consumption characterized by bone steaming, high afternoon fevers, cough, emaciated flesh, reddened complexion, thief perspiration, and a fine rapid pulse, use [the following]:

Qín Jiāo Bēi Jiǎ Sǎn (Large Gentian and Turtle Shell Powder)
from *Luó Qiān Fǔ Fāng*

biē jiǎ	turtle shell
qín jiāo	large gentian [root]
zhī mǔ	anemarrhena [root]
dāng guī	tangkuei
chái hú	bupleurum [root]
dì gǔ pí	lycium root bark
wū méi	mume [fruit]
qīng hāo yè	sweet wormwood leaf

These are not essentially different from the established rule of enriching the yin and clearing heat.

Yang vacuity characterized by a cold body and aversion to wind, lazy speech, absence of headache, little appetite, cardiac vexation, generalized fever, and a large pulse lacking strength, indicate the use of [the following prescription]:

Bǔ Zhōng Yì Qì Tāng (Center-Supplementing Qi-Boosting Decoction)
Lǐ Dōngyuán's prescription

huáng qí	astragalus [root]
rén shēn	ginseng
bái zhú	ovate atractylodes [root]
dāng guī	tangkuei
gān cǎo	licorice [root]
chén pí	tangerine peel
shēng má	cimicifuga [root]
chái hú	bupleurum [root]
jiāng	ginger
dà zǎo	jujube [fruit]

This [type of fever] is commonly seen in the latter part of the evening and early morning and is therefore precisely opposite from fever due to yin vacuity. There is an aversion to wind and extreme aversion to drafts. Fear of cold means diminished warmth and is not analogous to an external affliction where thick clothing helps [relieve the cold]. This is why there is an aversion to cold. If sweet warming methods for abating fever are not employed, and dispersing methods are mistakenly used, there will be incessant diaphoresis, and if clearing cooling methods are used there will be hiccup counterflow affecting the voice. If methods for enriching the yin are mistakenly used, this will result in spiritual fatigue and clouding, and pasty stools and diarrhea.

Another category of fever is that of blood vacuity. Fevers due to blood vacuity and those due to yin vacuity are closely related. Yin vacuity fevers are predominant in the afternoon and gradually diminish as the evening progresses. Fevers due to blood vacuity will appear after any slight exertion and will lack a regular pattern. When they are mild, generalized fever will not be present, although the facial area will be flushed and burning

and there will be heat in the hands, feet, and heart with abnormal bodily
fatigue. Prescriptions such as [the following] are used:

Dāng Guī Bǔ Xuè Tāng (Tangkuei Blood-Supplementing Decoction)	
Lǐ Dōngyuán's prescription	
huáng qí	(astragalus [root])
dāng guī	(tangkuei)

Rén Shēn Yǎng Róng Tāng (Ginseng Construction-Nourishing Decoction)	
from *Hé Jì Jú Fāng*	
rén shēn	ginseng
bái zhú	ovate atractylodes [root]
huáng qí	astragalus [root]
ròu guì	cinnamon bark
dāng guī	tangkuei
dì huáng	rehmannia [root]
wǔ wèi zǐ	schisandra [berry]
bái sháo yào	white peony [root]
yuǎn zhì	polygala [root]
fú líng	poria
gān cǎo	licorice [root]
jiāng	ginger
dà zǎo	jujube [fruit]

Medicinals influencing the three channels of the heart, liver, and
spleen are emphasized [in these prescriptions], as the heart generates the
blood, the liver stores the blood and the spleen unites the blood. Also, as
the generation of blood has form and the qi lacks form, we speak of yang
generating yin. Therefore, although this pertains to the blood aspect, qi
aspect medicinals are also employed. Blood and fluid vacuity may cause
fright illnesses such as cervical rigidity and opisthotonos. Nevertheless,
the febrile symptoms generally predominate and are related to external
affliction. For instance, for strong convulsions use [the following prescrip-
tion]:

Gé Gēn Tāng (Pueraria Decoction)	
Zhāng Zhòngjǐng's prescription	
gé gēn	pueraria [root]
shēng má	cimicifuga [root]
guì zhī	cinnamon twig
bái sháo yào	white peony [root]
gān cǎo	licorice [root]
jiāng	ginger
dà zǎo	jujube [fruit]

For softening convulsions, the use of [the following prescription] is
indicated:

Guā Lóu Guì Zhī Tāng (Trichosanthes and Cinnamon Twig Decoction)	
Zhāng Zhòngjǐng's prescription	
guā lóu	trichosanthes [fruit]
guì zhī	cinnamon twig
bái sháo yào	white peony [root]
gān cǎo	licorice [root]
jiāng	ginger
dà zǎo	jujube [fruit]

Also for weapon wounds and trauma where the flesh is broken, sores which have broken open, external pathogenic contraction with alternating chills and fever, slightly clenched jaws, stiffness of the neck, and the bodily rigidity called "breaking injury wind," [the following prescription] is used:

Wàn Líng Dān (Unlimited Efficacy Elixir)	
from *Zhāng Chí Yī Tōng Fāng*	
dāng guī	tangkuei
chuān xiōng	ligusticum [root]
jīng jiè suì	schizonepeta spike
fáng fēng	ledebouriella [root]
xì xīn	asarum
gān cǎo	licorice [root]
shēng má	cimicifuga [root]
tiān má	gastrodia [root]
fù zǐ	aconite [accessory tuber]
quán xiē	scorpion
hé shǒu wū	flowery knotweed [root]
xióng huáng	realgar
shí hú	dendrobium [stem]

Another decoction, *Cōng Chǐ Tāng* (Scallion and Fermented Soybean Decoction) from *Qiān Jīn Fāng* containing *dòu chǐ* (fermented soybean), and *xiè bái* (Chinese chive [bulb]), may also be administered. Althogh these formulas are related to blood vacuity, they are, nevertheless, not used specifically in the treatment of fevers due to blood vacuity.

Finally, as for supplementation, of the many ways to treat febrile patterns in Chinese medicine, dietary hygiene is of extreme importance. In general, for external afflictions of heat it is believed that eating rice porridge, lotus root starch, and simple bland vegetables is a good idea and that slimy oily foods are contraindicated, as are meat and fish. This prevents an increased production of heat in the stomach and intestines. This [dietary restraint] should also be continued for a period of time after the fever has abated to prevent the continuous arousal of heat known as "relapse due to dietary irregularity." Nonetheless, treatment of vacuity heat patterns is not based solely on dietary contraindications. On the contrary, dietary therapies involving foods such as beef, mutton soup, chicken, duck's milk, cow's milk, chicken eggs, carp, and sea cucumber are commonly eaten [remedially].

CONCLUSIONS

In summary, the Chinese medical categories that organize the treatment methods for abating fever encompass many etiologies and illnesses. In this area of practice we have a sense of the abundant content of the medicine of our homeland. Aside from the administration of medicinals internally, there are external treatment methods for abating fever in addition to the administration of internal medicine, such as soaks and baths. There are also many kinds and types of febrifuge methods such as acupuncture and tuina and, if we compiled all the modalities undertaken, this cornucopia would be further filled.

As narrated in this essay, eight methods are provided [for the treatment of fevers in Chinese medicine]: those of diaphoresis, emesis, precipitation, harmonization, warming, clearing, dispersing, and supplementation. Eight parameters are provided as well, those of yin and yang, exterior and interior, cold and hot, and vacuity and repletion. The three disease factors and four examinations have also been emphasized. It is understood that the three disease factors, four examinations, eight parameters, and eight methods provide the foundation for theory and treatment in Chinese medical pattern identification, and thus guide practice. Therefore, it is not difficult to see how these can be utilized in an integrated methodology for the treatment of febrile patterns.

Differentiating between the two major systems of external contraction and internal injury is of primary importance. Discrimination of different factors of external contraction and internal injury, and also constant observation of the interrelationships and transformations that occur between external contraction and internal injury, is also of essential import, as there is an intimate relationship between bodily strength and function.

An appropriate plan of management can be determined based upon comprehensive considerations of this sort, including the development of the condition and the particular situation of the body at the time of the illness. It is this extreme rationality that fixes the rules of Chinese medical treatment. While all formulas are organized according to standards, individual medicinals must be used with agility, and experience must be obtained in the use of these substances in treating febrile patterns.

The methodologies for abating fever in Chinese and Western medicine each have their strong points; however, it is my feeling that Chinese medicine has a great deal more to offer, and in using similar methodologies, the Chinese medical formulas are also, by comparison, more comprehensive. For instance, the scope of use for diaphoretic methods that abate fever in clinical Western medicine is relatively small, being generally confined to *gǎn mào*[7] conditions. In high fevers, methods such as those that act to mitigate the symptoms may be used occasionally, but they do not have a great influence on the course of disease. [On the other hand, diaphoresis] enjoys a broad scope of use in Chinese medicine, not only for the amelioration of symptoms, but also for shortening the course of therapy. As such it is not simply a palliative treatment for high fevers.

Next, in the latter stages of febrile illness, the patient is frequently weakened and although both Chinese and Western medicine sustain therapeutic methods throughout this period, therapeutic methods within Chinese medicine simultaneously utilize treatment of the root to ensure a concomitant preservation of bodily strength, as well as achieving positive changes in the pathology. Similarly, although these therapeutic methods are superior, it is essential that exploration progress and that these investigations not be taken lightly.

---

[7]Trans: *Gǎn mào* is used for the common cold and in Chinese medical differentiations of symptoms associated with the common cold, for example, *fēng hán gǎn mào* is wind-cold common cold.

Naturally, it cannot be said that the Chinese medical methods for abating fevers have no shortcomings. In clinical practice, there are febrile patterns that are quite difficult to bring to a successful conclusion; however, Chinese medicine is capable of rendering medical treatment that [in most cases] is highly effective, especially in the early stage of therapy. We must amply develop our own strong points, and progress in deepening our research.

(February 1959)

Cough from External Contraction

The condition of cough is commonly divided into two major categories in Chinese medicine:

1. cough due to external contraction.

2. cough due to internal injury.

Cough due to external contraction implies the contraction of an external pathogen that gives rise to cough. Cough of this type will often appear simultaneously with symptoms of external contraction. Sometimes it will be the salient symptom. What follows is an exposition of the primary symptoms, diagnosis, and treatment of cough.

1. Etiology and Pathomechanisms

Cough is an affliction of the lung. The lung governs respiration, connecting upwards to the throat and opening into the nasal orifice. They meet externally with the skin and hair. The lung is the principal apparatus for the exit and intake of air. If an external pathogen invades the [lung] channel, it may enter through the mouth or nose, or it also may be contracted through the skin and hair. Once an external pathogen has been contracted, this influences the clearing and depuration of lung qi, producing phlegm turbidity, and also an upward counterflow of qi that results in cough.

Cough due to external contraction may also give rise to symptoms of the viscera and, if there is qi stasis, symptoms such as costal pain; or, if there is copious phlegm, nausea is commonly seen. Nevertheless these possibilities must be clearly discriminated and primary and secondary issues must be clearly distinguished. Costal pain and nausea cannot be understood as merely "liver illnesses" or "stomach illnesses." These require the use of the technical titles, "liver cough" and "stomach cough."[1]

---

[1] For a further discussion of the parameters inherent in the use of this terminology see Qin Bowei's earlier essay on liver illnesses.

2. PATTERN IDENTIFICATION

Cough due to external contraction will generally be initially characterized by a scratchy throat, followed by a dry cough and a subsequent gradual increase of phlegm turbidity. This may be accompanied by simultaneous nasal obstruction and drainage. There may be aversion to wind with a sense of pressure in the head and a slight fever. There may also be an initial aversion to wind, and a sense of pressure in the head with nasal congestion and drainage, followed one or two days later by the onset of a scratchy throat and cough, hoarse voice, and lassitude.

Since the nature of external pathogens varies, if there is a tendency toward cold, then it is referred to as ***wind-cold cough.*** If there is a tendency toward wind-heat, then it is referred to as ***wind-heat cough***. At onset the symptoms are similar and the principal discriminating symptom is the presence of phlegm turbidity. Wind-cold cough will be accompanied by a thin white phlegm that is easily expectorated. Wind-heat cough will be accompanied by pus-like phlegm that is yellow in color and is not easily expectorated, with simultaneous symptoms of dry mouth and sore throat.

Beyond this [discrimination] there is ***autumn dryness cough,*** which most often occurs at the beginning of autumn when there is a prevalence of seasonal dry qi. In this pattern there is dry cough and no phlegm, or phlegm that is thick, gelatinous, and difficult to expectorate. This may be accompanied by nasal dryness, dry throat, dry lips and, if the cough is severe, thoracic pain.

The pulse presentation for externally contracted cough is most often floating and slippery. In the presence of dry heat the overall presentation may be hot.[2] However, in the initial stages this may not be terribly obvious. The tongue fur most often presents with a thin white coat in wind cold patterns and with a thin yellow coat in wind-heat patterns. In the case of dry heat the tip of the tongue will be quite red.

3. THERAPY

In cough due to external contraction where an external pathogen is the primary etiology, treatment methods for dispelling the pathogen are primary. The location of the illness is in the lung and the lung qi must be diffused and disinhibited. In sum, the therapeutic methods are those of diffusing the lung and dispelling pathogens. Based upon the characteristic of this illness, the above methods may also be assisted by the use of methods for transforming phlegm and normalizing the qi. Once the external pathogens are dissipated and the lung qi is cleared, the cough is naturally suppressed.

Simply suppressing the cough should be strongly avoided, otherwise, the lung qi will become inhibited and the external pathogen will become internally depressed, phlegm turbidity will not be easily eliminated and the cough will intensify, becoming all the more frequent and severe. At the same time, since the illness is in the upper burner, the medicinals used should be light and floating. It is said that "[medicines for] the upper

---

[2] A "hot pulse" in this context is one that is rapid.

burner should be like a feather for, if they aren't light, they can't elevate."
Otherwise the intent of perfusing the qi cannot be achieved.

PRESCRIPTION ONE: ACRID NEUTRAL METHODS FOR DIFFUSING THE LUNG

This prescription is indicated at the early stages of cough due to an
external contraction. When it is not obvious if the symptoms are those of
wind-cold, or wind-heat, then this neutral prescription is used to diffuse
the lung and transform phlegm:

baked *má huáng*	ephedra	4g.
fried *niú bàng zǐ*	arctium [seed]	6g.
xìng rén	apricot kernel	9g.
bèi mǔ	fritillaria [bulb]	9g.
jú hóng	red tangerine peel	9g.
baked *gān cǎo*	licorice [root]	2.4g.

This is *Sān Ào Tāng* (Rough and Ready Three Decoction) with the
addition of *niú bàng zǐ* (arctium [seed]), *bèi mǔ* (fritillaria [bulb]), and *jú
hóng* (red tangerine peel), which increases the strength of the lung-diffus-
ing and phlegm-transforming effect. For an extremely scratchy throat,
add *pàng dà hài* (sterculia).

PRESCRIPTION TWO: ACRID WARM METHODS FOR DIFFUSING THE LUNG

This prescription is indicated for wind-cold cough with copious
phlegm, aversion to cold, or an accompanying low fever. It is utilized to
diffuse the lung and transform phlegm, while simultaneously promoting
diaphoresis to resolve the surface:

zǐ sū yè	perilla leaf	4.5g.
fried *niú bàng zǐ*	arctium [seed]	6g.
qián hú	peucedanum [root]	4.5g.
bàn xià	pinellia [tuber]	4.5g.
chén pí	tangerine peel	4.5g.
xìng rén	apricot kernel	9g.
bitter *jié gěng*	platycodon [root]	3g.
fried *zhǐ ké*	bitter orange	4.5g.
jiāng	ginger root	2 pcs.

This is a modification of *Xīng Sū Sǎn* (Apricot Kernel and Perilla Powder).

Zǐ sū yè (perilla leaf) enters both the lung and the spleen channels.
Aside from coursing and dispersing wind-cold, it aromatically transforms
turbidity. It is therefore indicated for the relatively severe symptoms of
external contraction of wind-cold and phlegm-dampness. *Má huáng*
(ephedra) may also be added to the prescription. Measures for acrid, neutral lung diffusion may also be incorporated into the prescription. *Guì zhī*
(cinnamon twig) (3g.) and *jiāng* (raw ginger root) (2 pcs.) may be added.
This formula then becomes *Má Huáng Tāng* (Ephedra Decoction) with
additions.

PRESCRIPTION THREE: ACRID COOL METHODS FOR DIFFUSING THE LUNG

This prescription is indicated for wind heat cough accompanied by a dry mouth or low fever. It has three effects: dispelling wind, clearing heat, and transforming phlegm.

bò hé	mint	3g.
sāng yè	mulberry leaf	4.5g.
chán tuì	cicada molting	3g.
xìng rén	apricot kernel	9g.
bèi mǔ	fritillaria [bulb]	9g.
lián qiáo	forsythia [fruit]	6g.
jié gěng	bitter platycodon [root]	3g.
raw *gān cǎo*	licorice [root]	2.4g.

This is a modification of *Sāng Jú Yǐn* (Mulberry Leaf and Chrysanthemum Beverage). If the wind pathogen is severe, 4.5g. *fáng fēng* (ledebouriella [root]) is to be added; if internal heat is severe, 4.5g. *huáng qín* (scutellaria [root]) is to be added. This illness will quite easily produce a red sore throat, and although *gān cǎo* (licorice [root]) and *jié gěng* (bitter platycodon root) are in the prescription, it may be necessary to add 2.4g. *wū shàn* (belamcanda [root]).

PRESCRIPTION FOUR: CLEARING DRYNESS METHODS FOR DIFFUSING THE LUNG

This prescription is indicated for cough due to autumnal dryness. In coursing the pathogen, the inclusion of methods for moistening dryness must be considered and this [method] is distinct from clearing heat.

fried *dòu chǐ*	fermented soybean	9g.
sāng yè	mulberry leaf	4.5g.
qián hú	peucedanum [root]	4.5g.
běi shā shēn	glehnia [root]	4.5g.
guā lóu pí	trichosanthes rind	9g.
shān zhī zǐ	burnt gardenia [fruit]	4.5g.
lú gēn	dried phragmites [root]	9g.
kǔ xìng rén	bitter apricot kernel	4.5g.
tián xìng rén	sweet apricot kernel	4.5g.

This is a modification of *Sāng Xìng Tāng* (Mulberry Leaf and Apricot Kernel Decoction). Autumnal dryness is related to a recent chill and, in general, we say that it is differentiated from dry heat. *Wēn Bìng Tiáo Biàn* points out, "if the qi of autumnal dryness is mild, it is dry and, if it is severe, it is cold." If there is dry heat, the prescription must be assisted by clearing and moistening methods, and if this is severe, *mài mén dong* (ophiopogon [tuber]) and *lián qiáo* (forsythia [fruit]) may be added. Nevertheless, the nature of this prescription is vastly different from that of *Qīng Zào Jiù Fèi Tāng* (Dryness-Clearing Lung-Rescuing Decoction).

**PRESCRIPTION FIVE: ACRID MOISTENING, BITTER AND WARMING METHODS
FOR DIFFUSING THE LUNG**

This prescription is indicated for a longstanding external contraction of cough which has not been cured, or a situation [of cough] that improves and recurs, with a scratchy throat and cough that, in the extreme, will be accompanied by panting [dyspnea] and facial redness.

jīng jiè suì	schizonepeta spike	4.5g.
jié gĕng	bitter platycodon [root]	3g.
zĭ wǎn	baked aster [root]	4.5g.
bǎi bù	baked stemona root	4.5g.
bái qián	cynanchum [root]	6g.
qīng pí	unripe tangerine peel	4.5g.
gān cǎo	licorice [root]	4.5g.
pí pá yè	loquat leaf	9g.

This is *Zhĭ Kè Sǎn* (Bitter Orange Powder) with additions. It dissipates external pathogens, normalizes the qi, and sweeps away phlegm. Its focus is on diffusion and transformation and it differs from formulas that suppresses cough in a more general way.

The dose of the above prescriptions should be based on considerations of the severity of the condition and the age and constitutional strength of the patient. Overdoses are inappropriate. Aside from these prescriptions, there are simple treatments for external contraction of cough.

The following simple treatment methods and single-ingredient folk prescriptions may also achieve a favorable effect. For instance:

1. For scratchy throat due to injury by wind that is producing a cough, use two [pieces of] *pàng dà hài* (sterculia) and drink three soakings of those pieces. Also, if there is simultaneous throat pain, add two *qīng guǒ* (Chinese olive) to the sterculia in the soakings.

2. For wind cold cough accompanied by aversion to cold and headache, use 6g. *zĭ sū yè* (perilla leaf) and 2 pieces *shēng jiāng* (fresh ginger). These are to be decocted and drunk.

3. For scratchy dry throat, cough, and feeling "out of sorts," use a decoction of white or green radish, which may also be eaten raw.

4. For a dry autumnal cough, core one pear and insert 3g. *má huáng* (ephedra) and 6g. *bèi mǔ* (fritillaria [bulb]). Steam this and eat it.

4. CLINICAL EXPERIENCE

External contraction of cough is a commonly seen illness that must be precisely diagnosed and treated in its early stages to avoid long term cough and injury to the lung.

In therapy for external contraction of cough it must be understood that [methods for] diffusing the lung and dispelling the pathogen are essential. For instance, if the cough is simply suppressed rather than being resolved, the cough will be prolonged and will increase in severity. Nevertheless, it is inappropriate to diffuse and dissipate excessively, as this will also cause injury to the lung qi, making it difficult to suppress the cough.

Following administration of medicinals for diffusing the lung, care must be taken to avoid exposure to wind, and if there is accompanying aversion to cold and low fever, [any further] diaphoresis should be minimal. Raw seafood or shellfish are contraindicated and one should guard against stimulating an increase in the cough [by ignoring this caution].

In the diagnosis and treatment of external contraction of cough, a discrimination as to the nature of the external pathogen is of principal importance and, in general, at the onset the use of cooling medicinals is inappropriate, since if cooling medicinals are employed, the pathogen will not be easily dissipated. At the same time a discrimination of the symptoms of the illness must be made. For instance, the early stage of pediatric measles belongs to a category similar to wind-heat cough, and senile phlegm-rheum illnesses are often aggravated by the contraction of a cold cough. Neither of these conditions should be mistakenly treated as cough due to an external contraction.

In the case of cough due to external contraction, there may be concurrent symptoms such as abdominal pain and diarrhea, and they may both be treated together or differentiated in terms of treatment priority. Some substances may be employed that lubricate the intestines and these are inappropriate if there is cough and simultaneous diarrhea. If the body is weak, the contraction of an external pathogen may easily cause cough, and patients with the above-mentioned [senile or pediatric] symptoms may also contract an external pathogen, resulting in cough. In all cases, the differentiation of patterns and therapy must be based upon [assessment of] the entire condition.

[It should be remembered that] cough due to external contraction and common colds and flu often appear together, and these categories may be consulted interchangeably.[3]

(January 1964)

---

[3] Trans: Common colds and flu fall within the category of *gán mào*.

A BRIEF DISCUSSION ON THE QUESTION OF SUPPLEMENTATION

People often ask their doctors, "what about supplementation if my constitution is weak?" People also ask whether it is appropriate to administer supplementing medicinals for specific problems such as cephalic dizziness, palpitation, or insomnia. It is my feeling that these questions are very difficult to answer. While there is no doubt that vacuity patterns should be supplemented, [we must always ask ourselves whether] it is or is not a true vacuity. In what aspect is there vacuity? To what degree is there vacuity? In the absence of an examination, a prescription and appropriate medicinals cannot be determined before there is a thorough understanding of a patient's condition.

We speak of cephalic dizziness, vexation, and insomnia as being generally due to, but not limited to nervous debilitation. Hypertension, a tendency to effulgence of liver fire, restraint of the spirit, or worry and depression, may all give rise to such symptoms. Since the etiologies differ, supplementation may or may not be appropriate. If supplementing therapeutic methods are invariably employed and these methods will fail to conform to "pattern identification and treatment," not only is this of no benefit but it may indeed, on occasion, be deleterious.

Vacuity involves a great many factors that in Chinese medicine are divided into qi vacuity, blood vacuity, fluid vacuity, and spiritual depletion and spiritual insufficiency. Therefore, in vacuity patterns the location of the vacuity should also be sought. [Ask yourself specifically,] "what is lacking?" This enables skillful and appropriate supplementation to be rendered. At the same time, the patient's age should be taken into account, as well as their constitution and the duration of their illness. The strength or weakness of the intestines and stomach, the season, and the weather at the time, must also be considered. Otherwise, general changes in therapy will not yield ideal results.

Beyond all this, and aside from weakness patterns characterized by a great loss of blood, vacuity patterns for the most part have a gradual nature. Thus the urgency of the situation must also be evaluated and the severity of the condition considered.

In the case of a patient who is severely debilitated, and for whom one seeks rapid improvement, herbal prescriptions tend to have large doses. There are also those who presume that supplementing medicinals must always be expensive and precious. They presume that the more expensive the medicinal, the more effective it should be, and they ignore the proper function and utilization of these medicinals. The result tends to engender undue excitation and an increase in the severity of the symptoms, or, on the other hand, the dispersing and transforming functions become hindered with resulting symptoms of oppression and slow digestion. This too is an incorrect way of utilizing supplements.

Supplementing medicinals such as these should be handled in the [above-mentioned] manner; and the habitual use of enriching and supplementing dietary ingredients should also be dealt with in the same way. For instance, in the case of edible bird's nest, *bái mù ěr* (tremella), *hǎi shēn* (sea cucumber) fish maw, and soft-shelled turtle, all these foods have enriching and supplementing effects. Moreover, they appear in the pharmacopoeias and our ancestors frequently used them in their prescription compositions. Nevertheless, both their nature and flavor differ from one another and they are [each] utilized in a distinct manner. How are they most appropriately employed? And, how they are selected?

Based on my clinical experience it is evident that bird's nest and *bái mù ěr* (tremella) moisten the lung and generate fluids. These are appropriate for cough due to vacuity taxation with blood in the phlegm. Edible bird's nest fortifies and is able to clear, having a stronger effect than tremella. *Hǎi shēn* (sea cucumber) and fish maw calm the essence and supplement the marrow, and are appropriate for seminal efflux and impotence. The *hǎi shēn* (sea cucumber) simultaneously functions to moisten the intestines and to contain the urine. *Biē jiǎ* (turtle shell) enriches the yin and downbears fire, being indicated for vacuity of yin with internal heat and weakness in the lower extremities. These varieties of supplementing medicinals have a common shortcoming in that when they are used in large doses they have a gelatinous, fatty nature, [thus they] are slimy and difficult to digest. None of them should be administered in excessive amounts and they are especially inappropriate if there is a weakness of the intestines and stomach.

The use of foods for long-term hygienic maintenance provides good therapy for vacuity weakness patterns. Nonetheless, the above-mentioned foods are relatively expensive, preparation is inconvenient, and they are not indicated for administration for an extended time. I consider the use of fruits as substitutes, such as *lóng yǎn ròu* (longan flesh), *lì zhī hé* (litchee pit), *qiàn shí* (fox nut barley), *lián ròu* (lotus seed), *táo rén* (peach kernel), and *dà zǎo* (jujube [fruit]). The nature and tastes of these are sweet and neutral, and therefore they supplement the liver, kidney, heart, and spleen. Wash and cook the ones that are extremely pulpy, and take one each day for breakfast and lunch. They have no detrimental effects and are of benefit for impoverished blood, depleted essence, and general debility.

Naturally, for general vacuity patterns, general supplementing medicinals may be chosen for therapy. For instance, for cephalic dizziness and flowery vision, *Qí Jū Dì Huáng Wán* (Lycium Berry, Chrysanthemum, and Rehmannia Pill) is employed. For irritability and insomnia, *Tiān Wáng Bǔ Xīn Dān* (Celestial Emperor Heart-Supplementing Elixir) is used. For cephalic dizziness and irritability with concomitant vacuity, *Rén Shēn Dān Guī Wán* (Ginseng and Tangkuei Pills) is used. All these prepared medicines are quite mild. As long as they are applied for the correct symptoms, administration will cause no adverse reactions, and when regularly consumed they will produce a gradual lessening of the symptoms.

As for supplementing foods, in the case of anemia, aversion to chill, and lack of internal heat, mutton may be eaten. For kidney depletion with recurrent debilitation of sexual desire, sea cucumber and dried shrimp may be eaten, as these can also be of assistance.

In a word, vacuity weakness patterns should indeed be supplemented. Nevertheless, treatment of vacuity weakness patterns should not depend on supplementation exclusively. However, we have a saying in Chinese medicine that "one should not supplement vacuity," and this merits very close attention.

In summary, for rapid recovery of one's health it is important to consider all dimensions, and in utilizing regulating and nourishing treatment methods one cannot rely solely on the word "supplementation."

(April, 1959)

A Preliminary Inquiry into the Life Gate

An important issue relating to [understanding] the physiology of the medicine of our homeland is [the concept of] *mìng mén* (life gate). The life gate is given serious attention in Chinese medicine, being recognized as the source through which life is maintained and, over long periods of clinical practice, prescriptions that bank-up and supplement the life gate have been used in the treatment of certain illnesses [where T.C.M. is] achieving significant effects. As a result of this [clinical experience], the issue of the life gate now before us merits serious examination both in terms of research and discussion.

This essay is composed of two related sections: the first is concerned with the physiology of the life gate and its relationship to each of the viscera and bowels; the second is concerned with the significance of the life gate in guiding clinical practice. Based on the wisdom and experience of our predecessors, I have advanced my personal views on which I hope the reader will comment.

1. THE PHYSIOLOGY OF THE LIFE GATE AND ITS RELATIONSHIP TO EACH OF THE VISCERA AND BOWELS

The life gate is the root of life, embodying the true yin and true yang. It engenders the circulation of qi, passing throughout the viscera and bowels, the channels and network vessels. The life gate extends to the brain and penetrates the bone marrow, reaching the four extremities, warming the skin and striations, and having a guiding effect in maintaining proper physiological activity within the human body.

The earliest use of the term life gate is in the *Nèi Jīng* where it states, "The life gate is the eye," inferring a relationship to the foot *tài yáng* channel at the point *jīng míng* (Bright Eyes). This use of the term is different from the *mìng mén* discussed in this essay. Nonetheless, there is a mutual external-internal relationship between the foot *tài yáng* channel and the kidney channel. Based on the fact that the essence qi of the five viscera and the six bowels pours upward into the eye, this relationship cannot be denied.

Generally speaking, the *Nàn Jīng* is the earliest recorded reference to
the life gate [as it is used in the present discussion] and it notes that the
physiological activity of the life gate consists of:

> . . . *providing the residence of the essence spirit, connecting the
> original qi, storing the essence in males, and connecting with the
> uterus in females.*

As for the location and form of the life gate, Lǐ Díng in *Yī Xué Rù Mén*
recognized that:

> *Between the kidneys and within the white membranes [(i.e. the
> fascia) located there] is a small spot of moving qi; it is the size of
> a tip of sinew and excites transformation throughout the entire
> body, steams the three burners, dissipates and transforms the
> water and grains, externally manages the six environmental
> excesses, and internally directs the myriad concerns [e.g.: all
> things] morning and night without respite.*

Although the *Nèi Jīng* says, "the life gate is the eye," it also states, ". . .
beside the seventh division [vertebrae], in the middle is the little heart."
This "little heart" points to the importance of our discussion on the location of the life gate. Our predecessors divided the spine into twenty one
joints [or "divisions"] and, from top to bottom, it is located at the fourteenth [such intersection] and, from bottom to top, it is located at the seventh [of these] intersections. On either side of that joint is the kidney *shū*
point and in the center of it is the life gate point. The *Nàn Jīng* also
states:

> *The source of the generation of qi is said to be the moving qi
> between the kidneys. This is the root of five viscera and six bow-
> els, the root of the twelve channels, the gate of respiration, the
> source of the triple burner; and one name for it is the "spirit's pro-
> tection against pathogens." This is therefore the root of a person's qi.*

The *Nàn Jīng* notes that the activity of the life gate returns to the spot
of moving qi that lies between the kidneys. Based on the records of the
three documents mentioned above, it is evident that very early in the
development of the medicine of our homeland, the myriad correspondences
of the life gate had already been recognized.

Since the life gate resides between the kidneys, Chinese medicine recognizes that the kidneys and the life gate cannot be separated, and thus
the symbol of the *Kan* trigram [☵] is commonly associated. The meaning here is that the short lines above and below represent the yin and thus
both kidneys, where the single long line between them represents yang
and life gate. It was Zhāng Zhòngjǐng who said:

> *The two kidneys are symbolized by the outer even lines of Kan,
> while the life gate is represented by the odd line within, the one
> connecting the two and the two enveloping the one.*[1]

The kidneys and the life gate can be seen as a single whole and are
generally called the "mansion of fire and water" and the "residence of yin

---

[1]"Even" and "odd" refer to the even or odd numbers obtained by the yarrow stock method of
consulting the *I Jing*. See: Hacker E., *The I Ching Handbook,* Paradigm Publications, Brookline, MA, 1993, for discussions of the various consulting methods.

and yang." There are varying ways of looking at these things; for instance, consider the statement in the *Nàn Jīng* that "the left is the kidney and the right is the life gate," or Lú Bó's assertion that "both kidneys are generally referred to as life gate." These, nonetheless, do not deviate from the basic pattern and in terms of the general aspects of the life gate's activity, these seemingly contrary opinions are not in fact at odds with one another.

According to Chinese medical theory, the kidney posesses the qualities of skill and strength. At the same time the true yin and true yang within the life gate also depend on the support of the kidney essence. Therefore, it is obvious that the relationship between the kidney and the life gate is extremely intimate. Nonetheless, the kidney and life gate are, in the final analysis, two distinct entities and not one. Furthermore, the *Nèi Jīng* points out that between the two kidneys is a small heart, clearly denoting two distinct entities, each posessed of a distinct form. Therefore, we may unite them as they are united in the *Kan* trigram. However, they may also be divided and, thus divided, the life gate becomes a single *tài jí*.[2]

Our predecessors explained the functions of the life gate by the use of three analogies. The first is that of a papercut lantern *[zǒu mǎ dēng]*, the movement of which is completely dependent on the fire within the lantern. If there is an effulgence of fire, the movement is rapid; while a fire that is only slight will cause slower movement and, if the fire is extinguished, there will be no movement at all. The life gate can be appropriately compared to the fire within the lantern. The sufficiency, weakness, or extinction of the life gate fire influences functions of the entire body and so the significance of the life gate is well suited by the phrase, "establishment of the life's gate." (See Zhào Xiànkě's *Yī Guàn*.)

The second explanatory analogy is that of a cooking fire *[zào dǐ zhī huǒ]* in a brick oven. The rice in the pot needs fire to cook. If there is a low fire, things cook slowly; if the fire is increased, things cook more quickly, and if the fire is insufficient, the rice will not completely cook. The nutrition of the body is dependent upon the essence of the water and grain of latter heaven and the primary importance of the life gate fire is to assist in their metabolism, therefore the life gate fire belongs to former heaven, and is likened to a cooking fire. Former heaven is essential to latter heaven.[3] (See Zhāng Jǐngyuè's *Chuán Zhōng Liù*.)

In the third explanatory analogy for the life gate it is likened to the threshold of a house, which is quiet and closed. It controls the true water of the yin, moving and openly inspiring the ministerial fire of the dragon thunder.[4] This is a nice likeness to a threshold posessing the same actions

---

[2]Trans: *Mìng mén*, whether referenced as the small heart, life gate, or the moving qi between the kidneys, represents Chinese medicine's traditional positing of a logical relationship between the individual's overall strength and ability and the strength of the qi-moving, warming, and engendering functions associated with the life gate. However, this depends on the essential qi associated with the kidney, and both the life gate and the kidneys are morphologically and functionally distinct entites.

[3]Trans: Here Qin refers to the former heaven and latter heaven sequences of *I Jing* trigrams. The later heaven sequence is derived from the former heaven sequence. See: Hacker, *op. cit.*, for a complete discussion.

[4]Trans: This is a reference to images from Chinese mythology that have been incorporated into the imagery of Chinese medicine. The Fire of Dragon Thunder is a synonym for ministerial fire.

of openness and closure (see Bú Bó's *Yī Xué Zhèng Chuàn*). Although these metaphors are unavoidably fanciful, their figurative significance [for explaining] the function of life gate is nonetheless profound and they increase our understanding that the activities of life gate are the activities of fire, as well the activities of yang qi.

Based upon the *Kan* trigram [☵], it is my belief that life gate is primarily yang qi, and I have come to speak of life gate itself as the "supreme ultimate" *[tài jí]*. The generation of the *tài jí* has a duality similar to the duality inherent in the true yin and true yang of the life gate, and naturally its relationship to the kidneys cannot be ignored. This viewpoint that the life gate is the *tài jí* of the body, lying between the kidneys, is also promoted in the *Lèi Jīng*. Water and fire are germinated here, and water and fire are defined as the source of yin and the source of yang, as well as the receptacles of true essence and true qi. The yin essence of the life gate is the water within the yin, while the yang qi is the fire within the water. In his book, *Shěn Sǐ Zhūn Shēng Shu,* Shěn Jīnáo explains:

> The fire of the life gate is contained within the true water; initially it is not fire as fire, and water as water, separated into two entities.

In this way true yang and true yin are dependent and protective of one another, mutually generating and perpetuating one another as well; thus water and fire consequently aid one another. Therefore, although the activities of the life gate are most prominent in the aspect of yang qi, we cannot unilaterally emphasize the true yang while ignoring the true yin.

As for the relationship of the life gate to each of the viscera and bowels, Chén Shìduó, in *Suí Xuān Mì Lù,* explains them in this way:

> The heart receives the life gate and the spirit brightness is primary. It is the first to respond to things.
> The liver receives the life gate and engenders stratagems and considerations.
> The gallbladder receives the life gate and [controls the function] of decision making.
> The stomach receives the life gate and becomes capable of reception and assimilation.
> The spleen receives the life gate and becomes capable of transformation and transportation.
> The lung receives the life gate and governs the regulation [of qi].
> The large intestine receives the life gate and transforms and guides.
> The small intestine receives the life gate and disseminates and transforms.
> The kidney receives the life gate and there is vigor.
> The triple burner receives the life gate and establishes the sluice-ways.
> The bladder attains the life gate and receives and stores [the urine].

As to the activity of the twelve palaces, according the *Nèi Jīng*, the life gate is discussed as the foundation of activity for each of the viscera and bowels, and if the life gate sustains some injury, then the physiological function of each of the viscera and bowels will be influenced without exception. I have acknowledged this intimate relationship with each of the viscera and bowels with the following illustrative examples.

1. The life gate and the heart

The life gate lies between both kidneys and there is a mutual connection between the channels and network vessels of the heart and kidneys. The heart and the life gate are generally referred to as imperial and ministerial fire respectively, and the nature of these fires is that their respective qi strengthens one another. Therefore, the *Nèi Jīng* refers to the life gate as the little heart, and points out in addition, ". . . the imperial fire provides inspiration [*míng* (life fire)] and the ministerial fire provides executive [*wēi* (influence)]."

This illustrates the mutual connection between the life gate yang qi and the heart yang. Also, once the yang qi of life gate passes through the heart channel, it then posseses the ability to send the luminescence of the essence spirit through the entire body.

2. The life gate and the kidney

The kidney and the life gate are pressed extremely close together and the relationship of both has already been explained above. The *Nèi Jīng* also states, "The kidney rules the bones and the bones generate the marrow," and also, "the brain is the sea of marrow. The kidney stores the essence and controls the hibernation *[zhé]*, containment *[fēng]*, and storage of the root." Thus it can be seen that the products of the kidney and bone marrow, the activity of the brain, and reproductive vitality all have an intimate relationship. Furthermore, it is evident that the life gate plays an impotant role in these aspects via the kidney.

3. The life gate and the spleen

The life gate and the spleen represent former and latter heaven respectively. The generation and transformation of latter heaven is necessarily reliant upon the warmth and nourishment of former heaven's life fire. This is also discussed above. Nonetheless, care must be taken that the true yin of former heaven does not become deficient.[5] It must be continuously supplied to latter heaven. Therefore, Xǔ Shūwēi said, "supplement the spleen, and if one cannot, then supplement the kidney;" and Lǐ Dōngyuán subsequently said, "supplement the kidney, and if one cannot, then supplement the spleen," as a way of explaining the mutual relationship between former and latter heaven.

4. The life gate and the triple burner

The life gate is the source of the triple burner. Táng Róngchuān referred to it as the burning source, and the *Nèi Jīng* said that "[the triple burner] belongs to the kidney and that it upwardly connects the kidney with the lung." The life gate yang qi warms the interstitial striae and, via the triple burner, envelops the entire body. The constructive and defensive qi both issue from the lower burner. They pass through the triple burner and are generated and transformed by the triple burner.

5. The life gate and the gallbladder

Both the life gate and the gallbladder are aspects of ministerial fire. The life gate and the gallbladder have a similar character. The life fire

---

[5]Trans: the Chinese term here is *kuì fá*.

warms and nourishes the gallbldder fire, which causes the qi of the liver organ, which pertains to spring, to be uninhibited. It is for this reason that our predecessors considered the gallbladder the center of righteousness and that they also held that all the other eleven viscera and bowels are dependent on the gallbladder.

6. The life gate and the governing vessel

The governing vessel rules the body's yang. The route that the yang follows, according to the *Yíng Qì Piān* [chapter] in the *Nèi Jīng* [is as follows] :

> *The twelve channels begin with the lung, and ultimately connect to the liver. They connect to the conception vessel and the governing vessel as well. [The channels] do not necessarily reconnect to the conception vessel but begin another cycle with the lung.*

The *Gǔ Kōng Lùn* points out that the governing vessel pertains to the kidney, is joined with the bladder, and passes through the spine upward to the brain. This is how the text explains the area over which the governing vessel circulates and the fact that the life gate yang qi is transmitted to the twelve channels via the governing vessel. At the same time, it [the life gate] has an intimate relationship with the brain and kidney via the governing vessel, as well as a relationship to qi transformation within the bladder.

Because of this the relationships of the functions of life gate to the structure and organization of the viscera and bowels are conceptualized [as shown] in the chart below. As can be seen from the chart, the life gate yang qi is, in the previously-mentioned manner, related to each of the channels and network vessels of the viscera and bowels, and [the life gate *qì*] is transmitted to the entire body. [The life gate *qì*] is related to the organization of the internal viscera and thus they do not function alone, for instance the brain, heart, kidneys, and governing vessel are all intimately related [as are the other viscera and bowels], etc. In clinical practice there are many different therapeutic methods used for each of these.

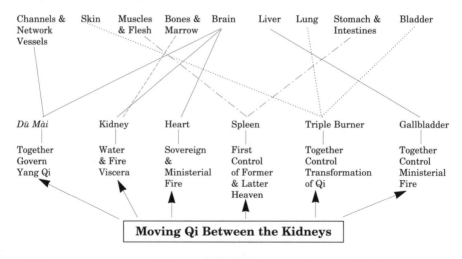

THE SIGNIFICANCE OF THE LIFE GATE IN GUIDING CLINICAL PRACTICE

The importance of the life gate is recognized in Chinese medicine and, in clinical practice, enrichment and nourishment provide the basis for its treatment. Because the life gate envelops and contains the true yin and the true yang, both of these exist as an integrated unit [within the context of the life gate]. Clearing and supplementing and warming supplemention are distinguished as separate techniques. In clearing and supplementing the middle burner there must be yang within the yin, because nourishing the yang is the foundation for enriching the yin. Similarly, when warming the yang, there must be yin within the yang, because nourishing the yin is the foundation for supporting the yang. Even if the true yin and the true yang both lose their equilibrium, producing a partially exuberant condition of both cold and heat, we must apply the techniques of balancing the yin and secreting the yang to restore health. One cannot simply use acrid warm or bitter cold medicinals to palliate symptoms.

The two prescriptions, *Liù Wèi Dì Huáng Wán* (Six-Ingredient Rehmannia Pill) and *Fù Guì Bā Wèi Wán [Guì Fu Bā Wèi Wán]* (Aconite and Cinnamon Bark Eight-Ingredient Pill) are frequently employed [for life gate conditions].

Liù Wèi Dì Huáng Wán (Six-Ingredient Rehmannia Pill)	
shú dì huáng	cooked rehmannia [root]
shān zhū yú	cornus [fruit]
shān yào	dioscorea [root]
mǔ dān pí	moutan [root bark]
zé xiè	alisma [tuber]
fú líng	poria

Liù Wèi Dì Huáng Wán incorporates [the above medicinals] to treat a depletion of kidney water, with head and eye dizziness, soreness and frailty of the lumbar region and legs, yin vacuity engendering fire, spontaneous sweats, thief sweats, emaciation, and lassitude. *Guì Fù Bā Wèi Wán* (Cinnamon Bark and Aconite Eight-Ingredient Pill) adds *fù zǐ* (aconite accessory tuber) and *ròu guì* (cinnamon bark) to Six-Ingredient Rehmannia Pill to treat a weakness of life gate fire and to engender earth for vacuity cold of the stomach, spleen, lack of appetite, soft stools, or chill of the lower source with soreness and pain of the lower abdomen, and so forth. All these methods conform to the principle of treating vacuity weakness of the true yin and true yang. Zhāng Jǐngyuè added [his observation] that Xuē Lìzhāi typically used Cinnamon Bark and Aconite Eight-Ingredient Pill to augment fire, and Six-Ingredient Rehmannia Pill to strengthen water to good effect. On the basis of the significance of these two prescriptions, *Zuǒ Guī Yǐn* (Left-Restoring [Kidney Yin] Beverage), *Yòu Guī Yǐn* (Right-Restoring [Life Gate] Beverage), *Zuǒ Guī Wán* (Left-Restoring [Kidney Yin] Pill), and *Yòu Guī Wán* (Right-Restoring [Kidney Yin] Pill) are the primary prescriptions used for the treatment of weakness and frailty of the life gate true yin and true yang. The composition of the four prescriptions is charted below:

Formula	Zuǒ Guī Yǐn	Zuǒ Guī Wán	Yòu Guī Yǐn	Yòu Guī Wán
Substance				
shú dì huáng cooked rehmannia [root]	Yes	Yes	Yes	Yes
shān zhū yú cornus [fruit]	Yes	Yes	Yes	Yes
shān yào dioscorea [root]	Yes	Yes	Yes	Yes
gǒu qǐ zǐ lycium [berry]	Yes	Yes	Yes	No
zhì gān cǎo mix-fried licorice [root]	-	No	Yes	No
tù sī zǐ cuscuta [seed]	No	Yes	No	Yes
lù jiǎo jiāo deerhorn glue	No	Yes	No	Yes
guī bǎn tortoise plastron	No	Yes	No	No
niú xī achyranthes [root]	No	Yes	No	No
fù zǐ aconite [accessory tuber]	No	No	Yes	Yes
ròu guì cinnamon bark	No	No	Yes	Yes
dāng guī tangkuei	No	No	No	Yes
dù zhòng eucommia [bark]	No	No	Yes	Yes
fú líng poria	Yes	No	No	No

Obviously the *Liù Wèi [Dì Huáng Wán]* and *[Gù Fù] Bā Wèi [Wan]* prescriptions are the foundation of Zhāng Jǐngyuè's four *Zuǒ Guī* and *Yòu Guī* prescriptions, and it is also appropriate to add *guī bǎn* (tortoise plastron), *lù jiǎo jiāo* (deerhorn glue), *gǒu qǐ zǐ* (lycium [berry]), *tù sī zǐ* (cuscuta [seed]), *dāng guī* (tangkuei), *dù zhòng* (eucommia [bark]), and *niú xī* (achyranthes [root]) to nourish the yin and support the yang.

We ought to recognize that in comparing the strength of the medicinals in these prescriptions in treating weakness of the life gate true yin or true yang, the *Zǒu Guī* and *Yòu Guī* prescriptions go a step further than *Liù Wèi* and *Bā Wèi*. The principles for the use of these medicinals are definitely a step toward a higher level of practice. Particularly because supporting the yang is not separate from nourishing the yin and, on the other hand, when enriching the yin, support of the yang should in all respects be given consideration, the inclination toward the use of acrid warm to supplement fire and bitter cold to drain fire is very inspiring.

What follows is a discussion on the value of life gate in guiding clinical practice based on my own clinical experience, which, of course, is not very comprehensive. For instance, in our treatment of spinal myelitis, we consider the primary symptoms to be paralysis of the lower extremities, or a sinking heaviness that makes it difficult to walk, a flaccid weakness of the sinew and bone, numbness of the flesh, lassitude of the entire body, lack of warmth in the four extremities, a cold chill in the lumbar region and knees, impotence, obstructed elimination or incontinence, and so on. These symptoms pertain to the categories of dual vacuity of liver and kidney, weakness of the life gate fire, and a loss of warming penetration of the yang qi of the governing vessel. Therefore, warming and supplementing the kidney life [gate] is primary, assisted by principles for extinguishing wind, quickening channels and arresting pain. [In this case] use *Dì Huáng Yín Zǐ* (Rehmannia Drink) with modifications and within a short period the symptoms will dissappear or gradually diminish and the patient will become ambulatory either with support or unaided.

Dì Huáng Yín Zǐ (Rehmannia Drink)	
shú dì huáng	cooked rehmannia [root]
shān zhū yú	cornus [fruit]
ròu cōng róng	cistanche [stem]
fù zǐ	aconite [accessory tuber]
ròu guì	cinnamon bark
bā jǐ tiān	morinda [root]
mài mén dōng	ophiopogon [tuber]
shí hú	dendrobium [stem]

[These medicinals] have the effects of being nourishing but not slimy, warm but not drying, and are capable of supplementing the lower source. Based on this experience, I use *[Dì Huáng Yín Zǐ]* in my treatment of Fredrich's ataxia presenting with symptoms of staggering and low tolerance for activity, as well as symptoms such as thoracic oppression, perspiration of the head, rough voice, hoarse gravelly voice, and choking with ingestion of food and drink. These symptoms all fall within the category of vacuity chill of the lower source, and an upward harassment of vacuity wind. With concurrent symptoms of muteness, I use the above prescription, with the addition of *yuǎn zhì* (polygala [root]) and *shí chāng pú* (acorus [root]) to perfuse the heart qi and to promote a rapid medicinal effect.

Chronic nephritis is an obstinate illness. Our [understanding of this disease] is based on the *Nèi Jīng*:

> The kidney is the gate of the stomach, and if it is inhibited, there will be an accumulation of water and similar symptoms; this will overflow into the skin both above and below, resulting in swelling.

Therefore, the treatment often proceeds from warming and supplementing the life gate to assist the transformation of qi and also strengthening the middle burner and fortifying the functions of transportation of dampness and turbidity. We commonly employ *Jīn Guì Shèn Qī Wán* (Golden Coffer Kidney Qi Pill) combined with *Wèi Líng Tāng* (Stomach-Calming Poria (Hoelen) Five Decoction), [because these prescriptions] take into account both the root cause and the symptom so as to achieve a satisfactory result. It can be seen that the dynamics of Chinese medical therapy in the warming and nourishment of the life gate, supplementation of the transportation in the middle burner, assistance to the triple burner, and the transformation of qi by the bladder, elimination of water and dampness, and prevention of accumulations, obviously entail a very different understanding of the disease than that of modern medicine.[6]

Incessant longstanding diarrhea, daybreak diarrhea, and frequent voiding of thin stools are generally spoken of in terms of chronic enteritis, and although [in biomedicine] this [term] pertains to illnesses of the intestine and stomach, in Chinese medicine we most often speak of treatment in terms of the spleen and kidney (including the life gate). Therefore, we typically use *Fù Zǐ Lǐ Zhōng Tāng* (Aconite Center-Rectifying Decoction) and *Sì Shén Wán* (Four Spirits Pills) to warm and supplement the life gate and to supplement the spleen and secure the intestines. This is referred to as the principle of supplementing fire and engendering earth.

Repletion panting [dyspnea] falls mostly within the category of the lung, while vacuity panting [dyspnea] largely falls within the category of the kidney. In terms of the kidney, we mostly use [the treatment] principles of supplementing the kidney and assimilating the qi with prescriptions in the category of *Qī Wèi Dū Qì Wán* (Seven-Ingredient Metropolis Qi Pill). Also, to eliminate phlegm rheum panting [dyspnea] in the lung, in addition to the application of *Xiào Qīng Lóng Tāng* (Minor Green-Blue Dragon Decoction), *Líng Guì Zhú Gān Tāng* (Poria (Hoelen), Cinnamon Twig, Ovate Atractylodes, and Licorice Decoction) is generally used to warm and transform the middle burner. If it is a serious condition, then this indicates the use of *Jīn Guì Shèn Qī Wán* (Golden Coffer Kidney Qi Pill) to warm and supplement the lower source. In practice, all the above prescriptions keep an eye toward the life gate yang qi. Therefore, if the panting [dyspnea] is extreme and on the verge of desertion with perspiration of the head, chills in the feet, and incontinence, which is indicative of an exhaustion of life gate yang qi, *Hēi Xí Dān* (Galenite Elixir) may also be used to directly warm the lower source and rescue it.

Of the clinical symptoms of debilitation of the essence spirit, the presentations of primary importance are insomnia, palpitations, cephalic dizziness, and inability to concentrate. The Chinese medical discrimination of patterns does not separate the two channels of the heart and liver. Because the heart and the liver are both related to kidney *míng* [*mèn*], besides nourishing the heart and liver, [treatment must] go one step further and concurrently enrich the yin to nourish the liver, and free the yang to nourish the heart. Also, because the life gate is intimately related to reproductive function, in cases of seminal emisssion and impotence occurring within the context of a debility of essence spirit, Chinese medicine

---

[6]Trans: "Modern medicine" in synonymous with "Western medicine" in China today. Here Qin Bowei is making a general observation about the fundamental differences in the basic perspectives of Chinese and Western medicine. His earlier observations using the example of hiccups focused on a specific aspect of this dichotomy. While a medicinal may affect a symptom, the complex of signs and symptoms must all be considered to be truly practicing Chinese medicine.

typically uses the term "kidney depletion" to refer to a dual vacuity of yin and yang. For the comparatively obstinate situations discussed below, in addition to enriching the yin and securing the essence, the principles of warming and nourishing the lower source should also be adopted. The case histories of Qí Yǒutáng also contain *Qiáng Yáng Zhàng Jīng Dān* (Construction-Strengthening Essence-Invigorating Elixir) which uses [the following medicinals] to achieve a satisfactory result in treating impotence:

Qiáng Yáng Zhàng Jīng Dān	
(Construction-Strengthening Essence-Invigorating Elixir)	
shú dì huáng	cooked rehmannia [root]
mài mén dōng	ophiopogon [tuber]
bǎi zǐ rén	biota seed
fù pén zǐ	rubus [berry]
gǒu qǐ zǐ	lycium [berry]
hǔ gǔ	tiger bone
ròu guì	cinnamon bark

He also pointed out:

> . . . supplement water in the midst of using warming medicines; then there is no need for concern about disastrous scorching when fire arises.

This renders strength to the evidence in favor of our advocacy for the enrichment of yin as the foundation of upbearing and supporting the yang in the treatment of life gate yang qi vacuity.

On the basis of the theory that "the heart generates the blood, the liver stores the blood, and the spleen governs the blood," Chinese medical treatment of aplastic anemia, for the most part, tends to emphasize the regulation and nourishment of the three aspects of the heart, liver, and spleen. I personally am in concurrence with Western medical diagnostics in acknowledging that the bone marrow fails to generate the blood, but [I] go further, promoting the premise that "the kidney generates the bone and the bone generates the marrow." Considering that the patient is often cold as well, with [indications such as] a pallid complexion and a susceptibility to catching cold, which are indicative of vacuity yang, I typically make the warmth and supplementation of the kidney life gate the primary concern, with an adjunctive principle of supplementing the blood. Powders of *lù jiǎo jiāo* (deerhorn glue) and *zǐ hé chē* (placenta) achieve a good result. These treatment principles are also applicable in leukemia and severe anemia and have no ill effects.

I once treated an eight-year-old child whose thoracic vertebrae protruded, a condition that appeared to be a symptom of tortise spine. However, because the family members would not consent to the orthodox treatment using a plaster cast, in administrating herbal medicine I primarily used *Guī Lù Èr Xiān Jiāo* (Tortoise Plastron and Deerhorn Two Immortals Glue) dissolved and stewed in yellow rice wine, using *shú dì huáng* (cooked rehmannia [root]), *fù zǐ* (aconite [accessory tuber]), *ròu guì* (cinnamon bark), *xì xīn* (asarum), *bā jǐ tiān* (morinda [root]), *huáng qí* (astragalus [root]), *mài mén dōng* (ophiopogon [tuber]), and *bǔ gǔ zhī* (psoralea [seed]) in decoction mixed with the above stew. The intention was for the life gate to to reverse the pathological changes in the spine via the yang qi of the governing vessel. Within two months an unexpected and ideal progress had been achieved and in a half a year he was completely cured.

There was also a case of gynecological illness, with symptoms of scant menses, post-menstrual abdominal pain and inability to stand and walk, severe leukorrhea, daily lumbar soreness, a cold body temperature, lack of warmth in the extremities below the knees, sluggish movements, emaciated appearance, and sinking faint pulse. She was treated with many *jīn* of *Shí Quán Dà Bǔ Wán* (Perfect Major Supplementation Pill) with no positive changes in her symptoms. Further diagnosis saw the condition as involving an equal depletion of the *chōng [mài]*, *rèn [mài]*, *dū [mài]*, and *dài [mài]* and also determined that a yang qi vacuity in the *dū [mài]* was the primary etiology. The use of *shú dì huáng* (cooked rehmannia [root]), *shān zhū yú* (cornus [fruit]), *lù jiǎo jiāo* (deerhorn glue), *dāng guī* (tangkuei), *tù sī zǐ* (cuscuta [seed]), *bā jǐ tiān* (morinda [root]), *yín yáng huò* (epimedium), *qiàn cǎo gēn* (madder [root]), and *hǎi piāo xiāo* (cuttlefish bone) was indicated to strongly supplement the extraordinary vessels.[7] Following administration of these herbs she became more comfortable; a half month later, the chills in the lower extremities gradually disappeared. Then *ài róng* (mugwort [leaf] floss) and *zǐ shí yīng* (amethyst/fluorite) were addded and the prescription administered continuously for one month. Her menstrual volume increased and her complexion reddened; following the flow, there was no abdominal pain.

Menstrual illnesses are related to the kidney in many ways. It says in *Fù Qīng Zhǔ Nǔ Kē*, "It is not due to a surplus of fire but an insufficiency of water" and "it is not due to a surplus of water but an insufficiency of fire." In reality, all the above case examples are indicative of tendencies toward exuberance or depletion of the true yin and true yang of the life gate.

In addition, remember that the defensive qi issues from the lower burner and is capable of warming the borders of the flesh, filling the skin and fatty striations, making them open and close. If there is vacuity and insecurity, with symptoms of body chill and copious perspiration, then modified *Qí Fù Tāng* (Astragalus and Aconite Decoction) is typically used. Also, since the kidney and the bladder have an internal-external relation, if the bladder is unable to grasp and absorb, with symptoms of urinary dribbling and urinary incontinence, and with an emergent sensation,[8] modified *Gù Pāo Wán* (Bladder Securing Pill) is typically used. All [these prescriptions] equally stress the treatment of the life gate.

Conclusions

In summary, the life gate is a crucial issue in the medical physiology of our homeland. Very early on, our predecessors came to understand with meticulous precision the location, form, and function of the life gate, as well as its relationship to the organization of the viscera and bowels, delineating treatment principles and prescriptions. Based on the theory

---

[7]Trans: As the diagnosis is one of kindey vacuity within the context of the *chōng* and *rèn mài*, these extraordinary channels will be supplemented by supplementing the kidney.

[8]Trans: The sensation is that the urine is dribbling when it is not.

and treatment principles available for reference in the documents left by our predecessors, we may be guided in clinical practice, so as to achieve a satisfactory result. Ample elucidation of the life gate is at the present an issue that merits attention and study.

I once did statistical work on the category of vacuity in the *Pǔ Jī Fāng*, and this single class encorporates one thousand one hundred and five prescriptions for treatments such as securing essence, boosting qi and blood, strengthening of the source yang, strengthening of the sinew and bone, dissipating phlegm, regulating the viscera and bowels, treating chronic chill, augmentating hair growth, clarifying hearing and sight, regulating the lumbar region and knees, promoting appetite, augmenting essence-marrow, strengthening and enhancing the will, keeping the face from aging, prevention of facial deterioration, lightening the body, and promoting longevity.

This constitutes a third of the entire corpus [of prescriptions in that collection of prescriptions]. The use of *lù jiǎo jiāo* (deerhorn glue), *bā jǐ tiān* (morinda [root]), *fù zǐ* (aconite [accessory tuber]), *ròu guì* (cinnamon bark), *ròu cōng róng* (cistanche [stem]), and *hú lú bā* (fenugreek [seed]) to warm and nourish the lower source appears in more than three hundred and ninety five prescriptions, which amounts to over one third of the total. If the ingredients for generally warming and supplementing the lower origin, such as *gǒu qǐ zǐ* (lycium [berry]) are added, they comprise more than half the above[-mentioned] prescriptions. Within these warming and nourishing prescriptions, aside from those that tend to assist fire, there are an equal number that have some bearing on the enrichment of yin. Thus it may be seen that our predecessors paid particular attention to the true yang of the life gate. However, it is also not difficult to realize that debility and weakness of the life gate function is in actuality a most significant source from which symptoms of vacuity and weakness are [globally] engendered.

Our predecessors recognized that not only should vacuity weakness symptoms, including chronic taxation detriment and vacuity desertion from acute pathological changes, proceed from treatment of the lower origin, but all the methods endeavoring to promote longevity and retard the aging process also must lie in the regulation and nourishment of the life gate. Longevity theorists and practitioners in ancient times pointed out that essence, qi, and spirit were the three treasures of the body, and Lǐ Dōngyuán recognized this in his statement:

> The qi is the grandfather of the spirit, and the essence is the son
> of the qi, and the qi is the root of the essence spirit.

This is also referred to as the "cinnabar field" and the "lower sea of qi." Zhāng Jǐngyuè notes:

> The source of the transformation of qi resides in the cinnabar
> field. This is called the lower sea of qi and is where heaven's
> source qi is generated and transformed. If there is a sufficiency of
> source qi, then transportation and transformation will be normal.

Quite obviously, the "qi" mentioned in these statements is the life gate's movement of qi. The cinnabar field, the sea of qi, and so forth, are all references to the life gate, and it is not difficult to comprehend that the longevity masters are saying that "breath-regulating techniques" and "returning the cinnabar to the inside practices" are primary in the maintainence of health within the lower source and its generation of qi. Present day masters of *qì gōng* say that this can be initially understood in that it achieves a balance of yin and yang within the body and adjusts disorders in the function of the nerves. The movement induced by abdominal breathing promotes the circulation of blood and fluid within the viscera and bowels, improving the capacity for nourishment within the bodily organism. None of these functions may be distinguished from the life gate.

While I have cited historical documentation [in this essay], I have also advanced my own views based on my clinical experience, although obviously this is quite incomplete. To facilitate thorough research into and clarification of this issue, we must strive further in our observations, and utilize modern techniques to attain an even higher level.

(March 1962)

AN ANALYSIS OF CASE NOTES ON WATER SWELLING ILLNESSES

1. Water swelling illnesses most often involve the three viscera of the lung, spleen, and kidney.

The following points are of principal importance:

The lung rules the qi and the qi must circulate. (The qi cannot be allowed collect, but must continually flow freely.) This is called "moving qi *[xíng]*."

The spleen rules dampness and dampness must be transformed. (Dampness cannot be allowed to collect but must flow freely.) This is referred to as "transformation *[huà]*."

The kidney rules the water and water must be disinhibited. (Water must not be allowed to collect and must continually flow freely.) This is referred to as "disinhibition *[lì]*".

If the qi circulates, dampness is transformed and water is disinhibited; this is the normal state. Contrarily, if the qi does not circulate, and dampness is neither transformed nor water disinhibited, then water swelling illnesses develop.

2. [Pathological] changes in the three viscera of the lung, spleen, and kidney have an intimate relationship with the triple burner and bladder.

Therefore, for the triple burner, circulate the qi and disinhibit water. For the bladder, disinhibit the water. The following chart illustrates these relationships:

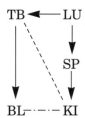

This chart allows us to understand the intimacy of the relationships of the three viscera of the lung, spleen, and kidney, with the triple burner and bladder. The triple burner and the lung equally rule the qi. The kidney and the bladder function to disinhibit water both internally and superficially. *Líng Shū, Běn Shū Piān* states:

> *Shào yáng [alluding to the triple burner] pertains to the kidney. The kidney upwardly connects to the lung and so [the triple burner] consequently supports both [the lung and the kidney] viscera. The triple burner is the granary of the central river and the waterways exit here relating to the bladder. . .*

The triple burner upwardly connects to the lung and relates to the kidney below. These three are intimately connected to the capacity for linking the water passageways and connecting them to the bladder below. Based on these theories the treatment of water swelling illnesses takes two tracks: one from lung to spleen, then to the kidney; and the other from lung to triple burner, then to the bladder.

3. Diagnosis and treatment of water swelling illnesses should be differentiated as vacuity or repletion.

1. The illness relates to a vacuity pattern if it has a gradual onset, originated in the face and head, and gradually moved downward into the lower body. [It may also] begin with the feet, moving upward, or it may originate in the middle warmer, causing a subsequent swelling in the lower or upper extremities before finally affecting the entire body. Vacuity symptoms, in general, most often originate in the viscera of the lung, spleen, and kidney.

2. The illness relates to a repletion pattern if it has a sudden onset, quickly affecting the entire body without being specifically located in the upper or lower parts of the body.

The lumbar region may be used as a criteria. If the swelling is from the lumbar upward, this [condition] pertains to the category of wind. If it is from the lumbar downward, this [condition] pertains to the category of water. If there is swelling in the entire body, there is an overflow of wind and water. In general, repletion symptoms most often originate in the lung, triple burner, and bladder.

ANALYSIS OF CASES

The case histories themselves have been omitted [but have been summarized below]. [First discussed are] two similar cases, both [of whom were] married women over twenty who developed their illness more than a year ago. Both had water swelling and, when their illnesses were severe, each had symptoms of vacuity desertion. Both patients also recovered from their conditions in a similar manner. (The biomedical diagnosis for both was chronic nephritis and uremia.) The two cases are contrasted below.

Symptoms	Case 1	Case 2
Edemas	Mild	Severe
Swelling location	Entire body	Entire body
Complexion	Withered yellow	Somber white (lusterless)
Spirit	Devitalized	Listless
Respiration	Weak voice	Rough respiration
Urination	Short, yellow; sensation of incompletion	Short, yellow; inhibited sensation (feels "stuck")
Defecation	Sometimes dry, sometimes sticky	Normal
Appetite	Poor, with postprandial oppression and vomiting	Anorexia, nausea, vomiting
Thirst	Mouth dry with no desire for fluids	Mouth dry with thirst
Sleep	Somnolence	Insomnia
Chills/fever	Aversion to chill Body temperature less than 37° C. Adiaphoresis	Elevated body temperature (~39° C.) Desire for fluids
Pulse	Slow, depleted	Floating, rapid, slippery
Tongue Presentation	Pale body Not slimy	White Little fluid
Other Observations	Visual dizziness, tinnitus Lumbar pain Cephalic dizziness Abdominal pain	Cephalic dizziness Blurred vision Confusion

These symptoms should be analyzed based on [categorization as] lung, spleen, kidney, triple burner, and bladder, as well as vacuity and repletion, cold and heat, in the following manner.

Category	Case 1	Case 2
Qi/blood Vacuity	Withered yellow complexion; spirit devitalized; weak voice; visual and cephalic dizziness	Somber white complexion, listless spirit; little fluid on tongue; cephalic dizziness
Yang vacuity	Aversion to cold; no fever	
Cold	Dry mouth No desire for fliuds	
Heat		Dry mouth; thirst
Absence of superficial symptoms	Tongue not slimy	
Presence of superficial symptoms		Aversion to cold; superficial fever; adiaphoresis; floating, rapid, slippery pulse; white tongue coat
Pathogens in the lung		Rough respiration; inability to lie recumbent
Presence of internal water	Short yellow micturition	Short yellow micturition

In comparing these two cases, it is quite obvious that the first case is internal, because of the absence of exterior symptoms and [because] the etiology is vacuity cold. Since the spleen fails to transform dampness and the kidney fails to circulate water, water swelling is produced. In the second case, although there are internal and vacuity symptoms, there are concommitant exterior and heat symptoms. Moreover, the tendency toward the exterior and repletion indicates that the etiology of the illness is in the lung, triple burner, and bladder, with the lung being the viscera primarily affected.

[These cases] are therefore similar in that they are "chronic nephritis," however, in relying upon a Chinese medical discrimination for treatment they are handled differently.

THERAPY, CASE ONE

PRESCRIPTION ONE: **Warming, transforming, and disinhibiting water: Warming both the spleen and kidney channels**

shú fù zǐ	cooked aconite accessory tuber	4.5g.
bái zhú	fried ovate atractylodes [root]	6g.
fú líng	poria	9g.
zhī gān cǎo	baked licorice [root]	2.4g.
dāng guī	tangkuei	4.5g.
bàn xià	pinellia [tuber]	4.5g.
chén pí	tangerine peel	4.5g.
shà rén	amomum [fruit]	2.4g.

Following administration of this prescription there was no change in the illness; then suddenly, ocular swelling developed along with a tendency toward suppuration; thus the prescription was changed [accordingly]:

PRESCRIPTION TWO[1]: **Clearing, perfusion, and bland percolation: Clear heat and eliminate wind, disperse swelling and disinhibit urination**

jīng jiè suì	schizonepeta spike
gān cǎo	licorice [root]
mǔ dān pí	moutan [root bark]
fú líng	poria
fáng fēng	ledebouriella [root]
huáng qín	scutellaria [root]
chì sháo yào	red peony [root]
mì méng huā	buddleia [flower]
jié gěng	platycodon [root]
lián qiáo	forsythia [fruit]
bái zhú	ovate atractylodes [root] burnt
chán tuì	cicada molting

Following the administration [of this prescription] the spleen and stomach were depleted, there was anorexia, nausea, and vomiting. The prescription was changed [accordingly]:

---

[1] Trans: Qin Bowei does not provide doses throughout.

PRESCRIPTION THREE: *Supplementing the middle and boosting the qi*

huáng qí	baked astragalus [root]
shēng má	cimicifuga [root]
dāng guī	tangkuei
bái zhú	ovate atractylodes [root]
chái hú	bupleurum [root]
gān cǎo	licorice [root]
chén pí	tangerine peel
rén shēn	ginseng

Following the administration of this prescription, the patient developed a cough and hematemesis. [As the illness exerted its] influence in the lung there was [a concomittant] appearance of symptoms of listlessness and vacuity desertion. [Thus the prescription was modified accordingly.]

PRESCRIPTION FOUR: *Supporting the origin and clearing the lung*

xī yáng shēn	American ginseng (powdered)
bèi mǔ	fritillaria [bulb]

Following administration, the bleeding stopped, although the spleen and stomach were still depleted [so the prescription was changed accordingly]:

PRESCRIPTION FIVE: *Supplementing the middle and boosting the qi*

[Prescription three was administered.]

The illness gradually improved, although in the last three days [while presecription three was taken] she vomited after eating, as well as spitting up a white frothy phlegm. [The prescription was changed accordingly:]

PRESCRIPTION SIX: *Downbearing turbidity and transforming fluids*

Prescription: 0.9g. *Yù Shū Dān* (Jade Pivot Elixir) three times daily.[2]

THERAPY, CASE TWO

PRESCRIPTION ONE: *Diffusing the lung and disinhibiting water; simultaneous treatment of the surface and interior*

bái zhú	ovate atractylodes [root]	9g.
zhū líng	polyporus	9g.
yīn chén hāo	capillaris	9g.
shān zhī zǐ	fried gardenia [fruit]	9g.
zé xiè	alisma [tuber]	9g.
fú líng	poria	30g.
mài yá	barley sprout (burnt)	9g.
běi shā shēn	glehnia [root]	9g.
chén pí	tangerine peel	3g.
bàn xià	pinellia [tuber]	9g.
jī nèi jīn	gizzard lining	9g.

[2]According to *Zhòng Yī Fāng Yào Shǒu Cì*, this is also known as *Zǐ Jīn Dìng* (Purple and Gold Tablet). It contains:

shè xiāng	musk	30g.
zhū shā	cinnabar	40g.
xióng huáng	realgar	20g.
hóng dà jǐ	knoxia [root]	150g.
xù suí zǐ	caper spurge seed	100g.
wǔ bèi zǐ	sumac gallnut	100g.
shān cí gū	shancigu [bulb]	200g.
nuò dào gēn xū	glutinous rice root	1320g.

Following administration of the medicine the aversion to cold ceased, however, the high fever did not abate and medicinals for draining the lung were added [as is described] below.

PRESCRIPTION TWO: **Draining the lung and disinhibiting dampness**	
sāng yè	mulberry leaf
dì gǔ pí	lycium root bark
zhú yè	black bamboo leaf
huá shí	talcum
tōng cǎo	rice-paper plant pith
xī yáng shēn	American ginseng (taken separately)

The fever gradually abated (to around 38° c.), but [the patient's] abdominal pain and listlessness were indicative of vacuity desertion [thus the prescription was changed accordingly]:

PRESCRIPTION THREE: **Clearing and moistening the lung**	
sāng bái pí	mulberry root bark
xìng rén	apricot kernel
máng xiāo	mirabilite
quán guā lóu	whole trichosanthes
bèi mǔ	fritillaria [bulb]
shí hú	dendrobium [stem]
lú gēn	phragmites [root]
xī yáng shēn	American ginseng (taken separately).

The abdominal pain gradually diminished and the stools became unblocked. Modifications were made to the basic prescription above [as described below]:

PRESCRIPTION FOUR: **Clearing and moistening the lung and stomach**	
xī yáng shēn	American ginseng
shí hú	dendrobium [stem]
xìng rén	apricot kernel
bái wéi	baiwei [cynanchum root]
bái máo gēn	imperata [root] (wild)
lú gēn	phragmites [root]
guā lóu zǐ	trichosanthes seed
zhǐ shí	unripe bitter orange
zhú rú	bamboo shavings (wild)
bèi mǔ	fritillaria [bulb]

After three days, there was urinary inhibition and constipation [so the prescription was modified accordingly]:

PRESCRIPTION FIVE: **Clearing and disinhibiting the triple burner**		
dāng guī	tangkuei	9g.
bèi mǔ	fritillaria [bulb]	9g.
kǔ shēn	flavescent sophora [root]	30g.

After the administration of this prescription, the situation was considered stabilized.

DISCUSSION

I am in essential aggreement as to the [correctness of the] treatment and prescription methods in these two cases. However, there have been divergent views propagated in the hospital discussion groups as to the [proper] course of therapy, since there were rather complex changes in the nature of these patients' illnesses. For instance, the second prescription used in the first case was *Bǔ Zhōng Yì Qì Tāng* (Center-Supplementing Qi-Boosting Decoction), and some people [in the discussion group] thought that *Zhēn Wǔ Tāng* (True Warrior Decoction) should have been used. I feel that *Bǔ Zhōng Yì Qì Tāng* supplements latter heaven in supplementing the spleen, while *Zhēn Wǔ Tāng* warms former heaven in warming the kidney (fire generating earth). In this case at that time, warming methods were not to be used. Because the hematemesis was of primary importance, the use of Center-Supplementing Qi-Boosting Decoction produced a relatively smooth and steady effect, although ultimately True Warrior Decoction would become the appropriate [prescription] to produce a decisive result.

[In] the second case, the patient suffered from constant fever, constipation, and occasional distension in the abdominal area. There are those who advocate the use of *Chéng Qì Tāng* (Qi-Infusing Decoction), while others feel that *Zēng Yè Tāng* (Humor-Increasing Decoction), *xuán shēn* (scrophularia [root]), *mài mén dōng* (ophiopogon [tuber]), and *shēng dì huáng* (fresh rehmannia [root]) are appropriate to clear heat and nourish the yin. I believe that this patient falls under the category of vacuity patterns [because there was an] absence of *pǐ* fullness or symptoms of repletion dryness that [would] warrant [the use of] precipitation.

Symptoms of urgent diarrhea injuring the yin were also absent, therefore, substances in the category of supporting the qi are not indicated. Furthermore, medicinals for nourishing the yin are for the most part enriching and slimy and, as this patient has a weak spleen-stomach as well as water [swelling], *Zēng Yè Tāng* (Humor-Increasing Decoction) should only be used with caution. It is best to use methods for draining the lung and disinhibiting dampness, assisted by *xī yáng shēn* (American ginseng) and *máng xiāo* (mirabilite).

Finally there is the issue of treatment of the root and treatment of the branch. As for case one, the simultaneous treatment of the root and branch is as follows:

Stage 1. Warming, transforming, and disinhibiting water is a root treatment.

Stage 2. Clearing, perfusing, and blandly percolating is a branch treatment.

Stage 3. Supplementing the middle and boosting the qi is a root treatment.

Stage 4. Supporting the origin and clearing the lung is a branch treatment.

Stage 5. Supplimenting the middle and boosting the qi is a root treatment.

Stage 6. Downbearing turbidity and transforming fluids is a branch treatment.

[As for} case two, this is entirely a branch treatment; nevertheless in treating the branch, the root must be considered. Therefore, in treating the branch the one must in all respects give consideration to the treatment of the root. This is related to the Chinese medical therapeutic method of treating the branch in acute situations and treating the root in chronic conditions.

As for prognosis, while there has been a turn for the better, vacuity patients present many changes and often suffer sudden aggravations, therefore one should not be too optimistic. Attention must be paid to the recovery of the correct qi, for as the saying goes, "if the correct is returned then there is life."

(March 1962)

QIN BOWEI'S CASE HISTORIES

Translator's Introduction

The following case histories complete the link between Qin Bowei's theoretical and conceptual discussions of Chinese medicine and how he actually expresses those ideas in clinical practice. The case histories included in this chapter cover a wide range of conditions, many of which Master Qin discusses elsewhere in this anthology. For instance, the case history covering wind water edema relates directly to his discussion of water swelling.

His case reports also reflect the variety of ways in which Chinese writers organize their cases. Many of Master Qin's reports consist of only a single case history accompanied by a discussion. Others, such as his case histories relating to cardiac pain and fever in leukemia, consist of a number of case reports that have been arranged to facilitate a comparison of the patterns involved, thus contrasting the various treatment strategies.

Note that the leukemia cases relate specifically to the treatment of fever within the context of leukemia and thus success is measured by whether or not the fever abated, not whether the leukemia was cured. This raises an interesting point in terms of Qin Bowei's perception of the limitations of Chinese medicine. His preference for an integrated approach to the treatment of leukemia, one utilizing both Chinese and Western medicinals, makes it clear that Qin was not a kneejerk ideologue who categorically rejected Western approaches. While it must be acknowledged that the integrated perspective was Communist Party policy during the 1960's, as it remains today, it is nonetheless a theme that is found in all of Qin's writings and is not merely a hollow bow to policy. Indeed, he has written an entire essay on the integration of Chinese medicine and biomedicine that was not included in the anthology here translated.

CASE HISTORIES

Case 1: *Li, a 60 year-old male*

One case employing modified Bài Dú Săn (Toxin-Vanquishing Powder) in the treatment of concurrent contraction of dampness, heat, and influenza.

Main Complaint: The patient had a weak constitution, chronic hypertension, frequent insomnia, and easily became tense. He had contracted a common cold within the past five days. One hospital had used both heat-resolving formulas and penicillin therapies and [after these treatments] the fever vascillated (between 37.8-39° C). He perspired copiously and this [symptom also] had not abated. The particular expression of the fever [in this case] was that it would become elevated at no fixed time and there would be frequent episodes of this [irregular fever] throughout the day. When the fever did elevate there would first be chills. When it dropped, there would be copious persipiration and aversion to wind. This was accompanied by headache, phlegmatic cough with difficult expectoration, lack of appetite, bitter [taste in the] mouth, a dry mouth with no desire for fluids, constipation, and short dark urination.

Diagnostic examination: The pulse was wiry, tense, and rapid, while the tongue moss was thick, slimy, and yellow in the middle [of the tongue].

Discrimination of patterns: The illness was due to an arousal of pathogenic wind, although there was also severe dampness and heat in the intestines and stomach as well.

Treatment methods: Since there were symptoms of intermittent chills and fever, lack of appetite, and bitterness in the mouth with constipation and dark urination, therapy was directed at the *shào yáng* and *yáng míng*.

PRESCRIPTION

chái hú	bupleurum [root]	4.5g.
qián hú	peucedanum [root]	6g.
huáng qín	scutellaria [root]	4.5g.
bàn xià	pinellia [tuber]	6g.
qīng hāo	sweet wormwood	4.5g.
jú huā	chrysanthemum [flower]	4.5g.
xìng rén	apricot kernel	9g.
jié gěng	platycodon [root]	3g.
zhǐ ké	bitter orange	5g.
fú líng	poria	9g.

Second Visit: Following the administration of one dose of the medicine the fever stopped fluctuating; after the second dose, it abated completely. Nonetheless, there was still copious perspiration; he [still] suffered from an aversion to wind and would cover up with clothing and quilts while sleeping. Consideration was given to the fact that while the external pattern had been resolved, the intestinal and gastric symptoms had not yet been eliminated. Moreover, the patient was old and weak, suffering from copious incessant perspiration and having difficulty sustaining his physical strength. The [treatment] plan was then changed to [continue] treatment with [the following]:

Guì Zhī Jiǎ Fù Zǐ Tāng (Cinnamon Twig Decoction Plus Aconite)

guì zhī	cinnamon twig	3g.
bái sháo yào	white peony [root]	9g.
fù zǐ	prepared aconite [accessory tuber]	9g.
huáng qí	raw astragalus [root]	4.5g.
bàn xià	pinellia [tuber]	6g.
fú líng	poria	9g.
chén pí	tangerine peel	5g.
gān cǎo	licorice [root]	2g.

Third Visit: Following administration of the first dose [of the above formula] the sweating diminished. After the second dose, the aversion to wind ceased. He continued to take the fragrant medicinals for resolving phelgm-damp and was entirely cured.

Comment: This was quite a complex illness. Of primary importance was the constitutional vacuity and the dual internal and external etiologies [that had] created a mixed illness. Such contingencies cannot be addressed randomly. Based on the initial diagnosis, the [first] prescription utilized methods that addressed injury by cold. Nevertheless, integrated in *Bài Dú Sǎn* (Toxin-Vanquishing Powder) are *chái hú* (bupleurum [root]) and *zhǐ ké* (bitter orange) to both upbear and downbear, and drain pathogens. This cannot simply be regarded as *Xiǎo Chái Hú Tāng* (Minor Bupleurum Decoction). The skill in the modification lies in this change.

Case 2. *Zhang, a 67 year-old male*

One case employing Guì Zhī Tāng (Cinnamon Twig Decoction) with the addition of huáng qí (astragalus [root]) in the successful treatment of a vacuity patient with an exterior contraction.

Initial report: The patient caught colds frequently, once every month or so, in endless succession. The symptoms were nasal obstruction, cough, hacking up phlegm, copious facial perspiration, and a slight feeling of fatigue. *Yù Píng Fēng Sǎn* (Jade Wind-Barrier Powder) was administered for a fortnight with no result.

Treatment methods: Following diagnosis, *Guì Zhī Tāng* (Cinnamon Twig Decoction) with the addition of *huáng qí* astragalus [root] was used. After administration of this formula, the patient became aware of a strengthening of his spirit and body. All his symptoms gradually resolved and and the contractions of cold no longer recurred.

Discussion: Throughout this illness, *huáng qí* was used in two [different] prescriptions. However, the results differed and the reason for this [difference] is quite simple. Cinnamon Twig Decoction regulates and harmonizes the constructive and defensive [aspects] and the [effect of the] addition of astragalus to secure the exterior is to strengthen the correct qi and expel the pathogen. Jade Wind-Barrier Powder treats the contraction of pathogens in vacuity patients in [those cases] where the pathogen itself has not been resolved. The intention [of this prescription] is to augment the qi and dispel the pathogen. In general, *huáng qí* (astragalus [root]) and *fáng fēng* (ledebouriella [root]) are believed to be mutually potentiating. Astragalus joins ledebouriella and there is no need for concern about securing the pathogen. Ledebouriella meets astragalus and there is no need for concern about dispersing the exterior. In reality, there is dispersion in the midst of supplementation and supplementation in the midst of dispersion. This differs from support of the correct and securing of the exterior. For this reason, if there are no superficial pathogens at all, administration of ledebouriella will actually provide an opportunity for exgenous pathogens to attack the body.[1]

---

[1]Trans: This is a rather obtuse discussion even in the Chinese. The point, however, is that in attempting to supplement the defensive qi, the exterior should not be resolved in the absence of external pathogens because so doing dissipates the defensive qi thus inviting an external invasion.

Case 3. *Zhao, a 23 year-old female*

One case employing Wū Méi Wán (Mume Pill) with additions in the treatment of longstanding diarrhea and amenorrhea.

Initial report: In 1951, the patient developed intermittent thin stools and diarrhea. Many kinds of both Chinese and Western medicinals were administered, but none produced a cure. In the early winter of 1961, the diarrhea became more frequent, especially at night, and the patient sought diagnosis and treatment.

Diagnostic examination: When examined she reported bowel movements two to three times per day, and once or twice at night. Before evacuation there would be borborygmus and abdominal distension producing pain. There was flatulence and frequent diarrhea which was unbearably awkward and embarrassing. A greater sense of comfort in her abdomen followed evacuation. This [increased comfort] was accompanied by copious perspiration, heat in the palms, dry mouth, a lack of appetite, lumbar soreness, and a sense of deep encumbrance in the lower limbs. She liked heat on her lumbar region and suffered from amenorrhea. Her pulse was deep and fine. Her tongue body was pale and the tongue moss was slimy and white.

Discrimination of patterns: The symptoms [were] related to a longstanding kidney vacuity: diarrhea, cold-damp, depressive heat, and binding hindrance.

Treatment Methods: Prescription methods incorporating Wū Méi-wán's use of acrid, sweet, and sour in combination to treat longstanding dysentery.

PRESCRIPTION

dǎng shēn	codonopsis [root]	10g.
ròu guì	cinnamon bark	5g.
huáng lián	coptis [root]	3g.
shǔ jiāo	xanthoxylum [husk]	3g.
mù xiāng	saussurea [root]	5g.
dāng guī	tangkuei	3g.
bái sháo yào	white peony [root]	9g.
gān cǎo	licorice [root]	5g.

with 18 g. *Sì Shén Wán* (Four Spirits Pill) (wrap boiled)[2]

Second Visit: Following administration of four doses of the [above] medication, the abdominal pain had diminished slightly, but what remained had not improved. Given the tongue coat which was white and slimy, it was decided that the deep accumulation of dampness in the lower burner should be eliminated first. *Bái sháo yào* (white peony [root]) and the *Sì Shén Wán* (Four Spirits Pill) were deleted from the previous prescription and *cāng zhú* (atractylodes [root]), *wū yào* (lindera [root]), *bái dòu kòu* (cardamom), and *pào jiāng* (blast-fried ginger) were added.

---

[2]Trans: Wrap boiling involves wrapping medicinals in cloth and decoting the wrapped ingredients with the other ingredients in the prescription. This prevents particulate matter from getting into the decoction and making it sludgy. Wrap boiling is also used to prevent drinking small materials that would be irritating if consumed.

Third Visit: Following administration of another four doses of the mediciation [as modified above], the abdominal pain had greatly diminished, the flatulence had lessened, and the nocturnal diarrhea had ceased. The tongue coat had thinned and the menses had resumed, but in small quantity and with a purple coloration. To the previous prescription *huí xiāng* (fennel [fruit]) was added to warm and unblock the kidney qi and [after administration of the modified formula,] all her symptoms resolved. In a follow up visit six months later she reported no recurrence of the diarrhea.

Comment: In this case of an illness of more than ten years duration, the symptoms of both daytime and nocturnal diarrhea with abdominal pain, encumberance of the extremities, and preference for heat in the abdominal region were indicative of vacuity cold in the lower source, thus pertaining to kidney diarrhea. Nevertheless, there was abdominal pain and distension, which improved following evacuation [and which was] accompanied by symptoms of heat in the palms, dry mouth, and amenorrhea. These symptoms were indicative of indigestion and loss of the transformation and transportation [functions]. This was accompanied by a concurrent presentation of liver vacuity and depressive heat producing a mixed vacuity and repletion, cold and hot condition, with cold-damp and binding hindrance of depressive heat. In this type of longstanding diarrhea or dysentery, Master Qin typically used *Wū Méi Wán* (Mume Pill) in treatment to achieve an ideal therapeutic effect.

DISCRIMINATION OF PATTERNS IN TREATMENT OF FIVE CASES OF TRUE CARDIAC PAIN

Case 1: *A 69 year-old male*

Initial report: [The patient had suffered from] intermittent precordial stabbing pain for more than a decade, which had become more frequent of late. The pain would radiate into the left shoulder and arm and was especially evident in the medial aspect of both wrists and elbows, thus creating a line of pain. This was accompainied by thoracic oppression, cardiac palpitations, and insomnia.

Diagnostic examination: The pulse was fine and rapid.

Treatment methods: The initial plan was to harmonize the heart blood and free the heart qi.

PRESCRIPTION

dān shēn	salvia [root]	10g.
yù jīn	curcuma [tuber]	6g.
hóng huā	carthamus [flower]	6g.
jú luò	tangerine pith	6g.
xuán fù huā	inula flower (wrapped for decoction)	6g.
shí chāng pú	acorus [root]	10g.
yuǎn zhì	polygala [root]	6g.
dà zǎo	jujube [fruit]	10g.

Second visit: The above prescription was administered for a fortnight and the frequency of the soreness and pain diminished, as did the intensity. Next, nourishment of the heart became primary, assisted by the regulation of qi and harmonization of blood.

PRESCRIPTION

rén shēn	ginseng (powdered, brewed)	1g.
dì huáng	raw rehmannia [root]	10g.
mài mén dōng	ophiopogon [tuber]	10g.
guì zhī	cinnamon twig	5g.
yuǎn zhì	polygala [root]	6g.
dà zǎo	jujube [fruit]	10g.
dān shēn	salvia [root]	10g.
hóng huā	Tibetan carthamus [flower]	6g.
yù jīn	curcuma [tuber]	6g.
xiāng fù zǐ	cyperus [root]	10g.
tán xiāng	sandalwood	3g.
rǔ xiāng	frankincense	5g.
sān qī	notoginseng [root] (powdered, brewed)	1g.

The above medicinals were modified based on the symptoms, and after administration for eight months, the precordial soreness and pain diminished from more than ten episodes per day to once or twice per day. The original stabbing pain was also then dormant and no longer radiated into the shoulder and back. Previously, there had been taxation fatigue, which required that he lie down frequently, but in recent months he had been busy at work and moreover had even been able to work a night shift. His complexion and sleep were also improved. Electrocardiographic revaluation of the blood supply to the heart also showed an improvement. When he had taken the prescription for three more months, *Dà Huó Luò Dān* (Major Network-Quickening Pill) was administered to assist in quickening the network vessels, as the elbow and wrist pain had not diminished. After more than ten days of continuous administration, [the elbow and wrist pain] disappeared and did not recur.

Case 2. *A 47 year-old male*

Initial report: [The patient had suffered] from precordial pain for one year. The pain did not radiate into the arms, although there was thoracic oppression and discomfort, and an incessant jumping movement in the left breast.

Diagnostic examination: The pulse was slippery and rapid and the tongue moss was yellow and slimy.

Treatment methods: The plan was to regulate and disinhibit the qi and blood of the heart viscera with the use of:

dān shēn	salvia [root]
wǔ líng zhī	flying squirrel's droppings
yù jīn	curcuma [tuber]
pú huáng	typha pollen
yuǎn zhì	polygala [root]
dà zǎo	jujube [fruit]
fú líng	poria

As there was a concurrent stomach illness, these were combined with:

zhǐ ké	bitter orange
chén pí	tangerine peel
shén qū	medicated leaven

Following four and a half months of therapy, the soreness and pain had gradually diminished, and *dǎng shēn* (codonopsis [root]), *shēng dì huáng* (raw rehmannia [root]), *dān shēn* (salvia [root]), *guì zhī* (cinnamon twig), *dà zǎo* (jujube [fruit]), and *lóng chǐ* (dragon tooth) were incorporated to regulate and nourish the heart qi.

After another four months of therapy the fundamental condition had stabilized, so powders of *rén shēn* (ginseng) and *sān qī* (notoginseng [root]) were used at doses of three *fēn* each, administered twice daily in boiled water for more than a year.   Based on the patient's own accounting, the stabbing precordial pain had been so continuous that he felt unwell most of the time, but this had now ceased and not returned.   In the past there would have been more than twenty episodes a day and now there were only four or five, and these were much milder in intensity.

Case 3. *A 53 year-old male*

Initial report: [The patient suffered from] palpitations [that] had appeared in the last six months and in the last three months there was also a drawing precordial pain with distending oppression in the thoracic area and with concommitant distension and flatulence.

Diagnostic examination: The pulse was slippery and rapid while the tongue was slimy and yellow.

Treatment methods: The [treatment] plan was to regulate and rectify the heart qi, assisted by harmonization of the stomach.

PRESCRIPTION	
dān shēn	salvia [root]
tán xiāng	sandalwood
yù jīn	curcuma [tuber]
shā rén	amomum [fruit]
zhǐ ké	bitter orange
chén pí	tangerine peel
zhú rú	bamboo shavings
fó shǒu huā	Buddha's hand flower
sān qī	notoginseng [root] (powdered, taken brewed)

The above prescription was [administered] for four months as modified based on the [patient's] own report that, prior to therapy, the pain would occur in cycles of two or three, with such episodes occurring several times daily. However, after administration of the prescription for three months, the pain ceased. Most recently, administration of the prescription was suspended for one month with a recurrence of only two or three episodes of pain. The [accompanying] sense of being flustered and the palpitations had also improved.

Case 4. *A 38 year-old male*

Initial report: [The patient complained of] daily precordial pain [that] had appeared over the previous six years. The pain radiated into the shoulder and arm and there was a sense of numbness in both hands. There were palpitations and a sense of thoracic oppression, postprandial discomfort, cephalic dizziness, and restless sleep.

Diagnostic examination: The pulse was fine and the tongue coat was thin and white.

Treatment methods: The plan utilized methods for nourishing the heart and harmonizing the stomach.

PRESCRIPTION

dǎng shēn	codonopsis [root]
dān shēn	salvia [root]
yù jīn	curcuma [tuber]
shí chāng pú	acorus [root]
yuǎn zhì	polygala [root]
dà zǎo	jujube [fruit]
zhǐ ké	bitter orange
chén pí	tangerine peel
sān qī	notoginseng [root] (powdered, taken brewed)

After administration of six doses of the medication, the cardiac pain gradually diminished, and the [patient's] appetite improved as well. The numbness in the hands diminished but the tips of the fingers were [still] chilled. The *zhǐ ké* (bitter orange) was deleted from the original prescription, and *shēng dì huáng* (raw rehmannia [root]) and *guì zhī* (cinnamon twig) were added. Once there had been an intial improvement, medicinals such as *lù jiǎo jiāo* (deerhorn glue), *mài mén dōng* (ophiopogon [tuber]), *bái sháo yào* (white peony [root]), and *hóng huā* (carthamus [flower]) were incorporated, and after six months the basic cardiac pain ceased.

Case 5. *A 43 year-old female*

Initial report: [The patient complained of] mild precordial pain, thoracic oppression, difficult respiration, cephalic dizziness, taxation fatigue, and somnolence persisting for two years.

Diagnostic examination: The tongue was clear, and the pulse was deep, thin, and weak.

Treatment methods: The [treatment] plan was primarily to regulate and nourish the heart qi.

PRESCRIPTION

dǎng shēn	codonopsis [root]
mài mén dōng	ophiopogon [tuber]
ē jiāo	ass hide glue
guì zhī	cinnamon twig
dān shēn	salvia [root]
yuǎn zhì	polygala [root]
dà zǎo	jujube [fruit]
yù jīn	curcuma [tuber]

Following administration of six doses of the prescription, the precordial pain diminished. Employing modifications [of the basic prescription] the symptoms clearly improved. After four months of therapy, other than a sense of taxation fatigue with exertion, the precordial pain did not recur.

Commentary

Based on my experience in the treatment of thoracic bi, the fundamental prescription to be employed is the established prescription, *Fú Mài Tāng* (Pulse-Resorative Decoction), which treats a binding regularly interrupted pulse, cardiac movement, and palpitations. It uses *shēng dì huáng* (raw rehmannia [root]), *mài mén dōng* (ophiopogon [tuber]), and *ē jiāo* (ass hide glue) to nourish heart blood, and *rén shēn* (ginseng) and *guì zhī* (cinnamon twig) to support the heart yang, as these fit the pathomechanism of cardic pain. Since the heart stores the spirit and sweat is the fluid of the heart, and because the root illness is typically accompanied by palpitations, copious perspiration, and insomnia, we may consider using *Yǎng Xīn Tāng* (Heart-Nourishing Decoction) with *Guī Pí Tāng* (Spleen-Returning Decoction), which combines medicinals such as *dāng guī* (tangkuei), *yuǎn zhì* (polygala [root]), *suān zǎo rén* (spiny jujube [kernel]), *wǔ wèi zǐ* (schisandra [berry]), *fú líng* (poria), *lóng yǎn ròu* (longan flesh), and *bǎi zǐ rén* (biota seed). However, it is unable to nourish the heart and calm the spirit as the primary thrust of treatment.

At the same time, we must attend to the soreness and pain that is the primary symptom of the root illness. As the primary etiology of this soreness and pain is inhibition of the normal circulation of qi and blood, how the obstruction in the blood flow is expelled and the free flow of circulation is promoted is the therapeutic relationship of primary importance. In considering quickening the blood, dispelling stasis, and generating the new, I initially use *Dān Shēn Yǐn* (Salvia Beverage) as the primary prescription. This prescription originally treats cardiac and gastric soreness and pain [and is prescribed] with *dān shēn* (salvia [root]), [which was] chosen because it enters both the heart and pericardium channels and frees the blood vessels. *Tán xiāng* (sandalwood) dissipates stagnant qi from the chest without the side effect of being acrid, drying, injurious, and dissipating. Beyond this, *wǔ líng zhī* (flying squirrel's droppings), *yán hú suǒ* (corydalis [tuber]), and *rǔ xiāng* (frankincense) from *Shóu Nián Sàn* (Instant Relief Powder) are also used to enter the heart and arrest pain. Nevertheless, based on clinical evidence, aside from the strong stabilizing effect of salvia notoginseng and Tibetan carthamus [these medicinals are able] to warm, promote free flow, quicken the blood, dissipate stasis, and stop pain, all to good effect. *Yù jīn* (curcuma [tuber]) enters the heart and is a qi within the blood medicinal. At the same time, it functions to crack stasis and generate new blood and, as such, is an important medicinal [that is] in common use.

In treating gripping pain, the three methods of nourishing the blood, supporting the yang, and quickening the blood are interrelated. The enhancement of cardiac function and normalization of blood circulation are of principal importance. Nevertheless, primary and secondary [goals] must be distinguished based on the entire pathological condition. At the same time, we must attend to the relationship of the root illness to the symptoms and their etiology, so as to deal with them in an appropriate manner. For instance, in a vacuity weakness situation it is obvious that nourishing the blood and supporting the yang is primary, as facilitated by *dān shēn* (salvia [root]) and *yù jīn* (curcuma [tuber]). In the case of frequent soreness and pain, quickening the blood is primary, facilitated by *shēng dì huáng* (fresh rehmannia [root]) and *ē jiāo* (ass hide glue). In the consolidation phase, crushed powders of *rén shēn* (ginseng) and *sān qī* (notoginseng [root]) are also commonly administered. When support of the heart yang with *guì zhī* (cinnamon twig) is primary, it is combined with *rén shēn* (ginseng). For instance, if there is recurrent cold, these [medicinals] may be combined with *xì xīn* (asarum) to warm the channels. Also, in cases of thoracic oppression connecting to the middle cavity, or in those [cases with a] tendency to postprandial cardiac pain, *xiè bái* (Chinese chive [bulb]) and *guā lóu zǐ* (trichosanthes seed) are indicated to harmonize the middle. For thoracic oppression and obstruction, with shortness of breath on the verge of expiry, *xuán fù huā* (inula flower) and *xiāng fù zǐ* (cyperus [root]) may also be added.

FIVE CASES IN THE DISCRIMINATION OF PATTERNS, TREATMENT, AND CURE OF FEVER IN LEUKEMIA

Case 1. *A female patient*

Initial report: [The patient suffered from] lymphocytic leukemia and had high fevers of 40° C. and above. She reported that in the last three months she had suffered from intermitent fever, as well as from taxation fatigue accompanied by a cold body, cough, visual dizziness, palpitations, retching and nausea, and dry lips.

Diagnostic examination: The pulse was thin and rapid and her perspiration was extremely copious.

Discrimination of patterns: The diagnosis was vacuity of yin with internal heat and that she was also harboring a recent [external] pathogen.

PRESCRIPTION

dì huáng	raw rehmannia [root]
biē jiǎ	turtle shell
huáng qí	astragalus [root]
shēng má	cimicifuga [root]
qīng hāo	sweet wormwood
sāng yè	mulberry leaf
mǔ dān pí	moutan [root bark]
qián hú	peucedanum [root]

After administration of three doses of the medication, the fever diminished and then [entirely] cleared.

Case 2. *A male patient*

Initial report: [The patient suffered from] chronic granulocytic leukemia. Every day towards nightfall a fever of 40° C. would arise and towards the second half of the evening he would break into a spontaneous sweat and become chilled. This dramatic [symptom] had been recurring for six months. He would sometimes have a slight fever in the palms of his hands, yet both feet lacked warmth. His lower back was especially sore and painful and he would defecate [only] once every several days.

Diagnostic examination: The tongue coat was thick and slimy, while the pulse was deep, fine, and lacking in strength.

Discrimination of patterns: The diagnosis was dual vacuity of yin and yang in the lower burner, and devitalization of central qi.

Treatment methods: The [following] medicinals were used, as they are sweet and warm, and eliminate heat:

PRESCRIPTION

huáng qí	astragalus [root]
shēng dì huáng	fresh rehmannia [root]
dāng guī	tangkuei
ròu cōng róng	cistanche [stem]
shēng má	cimicifuga [root]
bái zhú	ovate atractylodes [root]
zé xiè	alisma [tuber]

By the next evening the fever had cleared.

Case 3. *A male patient*

Initial report: [The patient suffered from] an acute episode of chronic granulocytic leukemia. He had had a cough for a month and for the past week had developed a fever each night. The fever would be preceded by reddening of the eyes, thoracic oppression, and shivering. The body temperature would rise to 41° C., there would be spontaneous perspiration, and it would [then] resolve. This was accompanied by oral dryness and short voidings of scant urine.

Diagnostic examination: The tongue coat [was] thick, yellow, and slimy and the pulse was fine, slippery, and strong.

Discrimination of patterns: The diagnosis was a pathogenic contraction in a vacuity body, joint hindrance of phlegm dampness, and a failure to expel and drain [water].

Treatment methods: [These medicinals] were chosen as methods for harmonizing and resolution, clearing and transformation:

PRESCRIPTION

chái hú	bupleurum [root]
huáng qín	scutellaria [root]
bàn xià	pinellia [tuber]
huáng lián	coptis [root]
hòu pò	magnolia bark
zhī mǔ	anemarrhena [root]
bèi mǔ	fritillaria [bulb]
jú hóng	red tangerine peel

The medication was administered in the afternoon, and by that evening the chills and fever had ceased. It was then administered continuously each morning and the strength of the fever also abated to 38° C.

Case 4. *A male patient*

Initial report: [The patient suffered from] acute lymphocytic leukemia. He had a persistent generalized fever, cough with sticky phlegm, a gripping pain in the right costal region, and a sore throat [which was coated] with white curd.

Diagnostic examination: The tongue coat was coarse and slimy, while the pulse was fine, slippery, and rapid.

Discrimination of patterns: The diagnosis was deep-lying heat in the lung and dual injury to the qi and yin.

Treatment methods: The [following] medicinals were used:

PRESCRIPTION

xuán shēn	scrophularia [root]
mài mén dōng	ophiopogon [tuber]
shí gāo	gypsum
zhī mǔ	anemarrhena [root]
bèi mǔ	fritillaria [bulb]
sāng bái pí	mulberry root bark
tíng lì zǐ	tingli
bái máo gēn	imperata [root]
lú gēn	phragmites [root]

The fever abated and the cough ceased.

Case 5. *A male patient*

Initial report: [The patient suffered from] acute granulocytic leukemia. There was generalized fever, heat in the palms of the hands, a distending pain at the temples and forehead, glomus and fullness in the chest and abdomen, oral putrescence and halitosis, constipation, and darkened urination.

Diagnostic examination: The tongue was slimy, and the pulse was large, slippery, and rapid.

Pattern identification: The diagnosis was lung and kidney vacuity yin and accumulation of damp-heat in the intestines and stomach.

Treatment methods: The [following] medicinals were used:

PRESCRIPTION

xī yáng shēn	American ginseng
běi shā shēn	glehnia [root]
zhī mǔ	anemarrhena [root]
pèi lán	eupatorium
shān zhī zǐ	gardenia [fruit]
lú huì	aloe

[The aloe was] administered separately to clear heat and guide stasis [outward]. After administration of the medication, the stools became smooth, the chest and abdomen gradually relaxed, and the generalized fever normalized.

Commentary

In these cases it is evident that the mechanisms at work in leukemic fevers are fairly complex. Therapy is based upon a Chinese medical pattern identification and, despite the predominantly poor prognosis in this illness, a temporary amelioration of the patient's suffering can be achieved. In leukemia combined with external contractions such as pneumonia, medicinals such as *má huáng* (ephedra), *xìng rén* (apricot kernel), *shí gāo* (gypsum), *sāng bái pí* (mulberry root bark), *zhī mǔ* (anemarrhena [root]), *bèi mǔ* (fritillaria [bulb]), and *lú gēn* (phragmites [root]) may be used.

Pneumonia may also transform to pulmonary abcess, in which case medicinals such as *chì sháo yào* (red peony [root]), *bái sháo yào* (white peony [root]), *bài jiàng cǎo* (baijiang), *mǔ dān pí* (moutan [root bark]), *táo rén* (peach kernel), *yǐ rén* coix [seed], *dōng guā zǐ* (wax gourd seed), and *lú gēn* (phragmites [root]) may be used. Pathological changes such as open sores in the oral cavity, throat, or the sides of the upper palate are common appearances in leukemia and pertain to the categories of oral gan and oral putrescence. These are primarily due to injury to stomach yin, upflaming of vacuity fire, or vacuity of kidney yin with upfloating of vacuity fire. *Shí hú* (dendrobium [stem]), *dì huáng* (rehmannia [root]), *xuán shēn* (scrophularia [root]), and *mài mén dōng* (ophiopogon [tuber]) are used initially, [with treatment] progressing to incorporate *ròu guì* (cinnamon bark) to guide the fire back to the source, and the topical application of *Qīng Dài Sǎn* (Indigo Powder) to clear heat and resolve toxins.

The symptomology of leukemia is complex; its transformations are rapid and prone to relapse with dire consequences. I incorporate a combination of Chinese and Western medicine [in patients' treatment], giving consideration to the [patient's] constitution and basing treatment on the pattern, thereby realizing some success. However, continuous experience is still required.

FOUR CASES IN THE DISCRIMINATION OF PATTERNS, TREATMENT, AND CURE OF WATER DISTURBANCE

Case 1: *Wang, a 28 year-old female*

One case on the use of tailored Fáng Jǐ Fú Líng Tāng (Fangji and Poria (Hoelen) Decoction) in the treatment and cure of skin water.

Initial report: For one year the patient had suffered from persistent edematous swelling which would sometimes be mild and sometimes severe. Western diuretic medications had been used as had Chinese medicinals employing methods to strengthen the spleen, warm the kidney, induce diaphoresis, and disinhibit urination; however, there was no obvious effect. [It was at this stage that] I was called for consultation.

Diagnostic examination: At that time it could be seen that there was edematous swelling in the entire body, the abdomen was bloated all over, the back was rough, and her urination was short and yellow. The pulse was wiry and slippery, while the tongue was tender and red, with a thin white coat. There were no signs of a vacuity of spleen and kidney yang. Further examination revealed that the enlarged abdomen was not hard upon palpation, there was no thoracic or diaphragmatic oppression, she had an appetite, and there was no postprandial distension. She had one bowel movement per day and suffered from very little flatulence.

Discrimination of patterns: The explanation [for her condition] was that the water was not in the interior but in the flesh of the exterior. This was decidedly "skin water."

Treatment methods: Tailored *Fáng Jǐ Fú Líng Tāng* (Fangji and Poria (Hoelen) Decoction), was used for treatment:

PRESCRIPTION		
hàn fáng jǐ	northern fangji [root]	15g.
huáng qí	astragalus [root]	15g.
fú líng pí	poria skin	15g.
guì zhī	cinnamon twig	6g.
gān cǎo	licorice [root]	3g.
shēng jiāng	fresh ginger	2pcs.
dà zǎo	jujube	3pcs.

After administration of two doses of the medication, the [patient's volume of] urine gradually increased. The source prescription was modified and in a fortnight the symptoms had completely disappeared.

Commentary

"Wind water" and "skin water" are two patterns [that are both] associated with water in the flesh. However, wind water is associated with an external contraction of wind-cold and skin water is not. Based on the particulars of this case it was without a doubt skin water. The [treatment] plan was therefore not to use *Má Huáng Jiā Zhú Tāng* (Ephedra Decoction Plus Ovate Atractylodes) and *Yuè Bì Jiā Zhú Tāng* (Spleen-Effusing Decoction Plus Ovate Atractylodes) to promote diaphoresis and disinhibit water, but to use *Fáng Jǐ Fú Líng Tang* (Fangji and Poria (Hoelen) Decoction) to circulate the qi and disinhibit urination. Master Qin believed that although diaphoretic methods could be used in skin water [cases], the condition was already chronic and it was inappropriate to further injure the defense qi. In applying Fangji and Poria (Hoelen) Decoction, the *huáng qí* (astragalus [root]) was used to assist the *yī wén qián* (graciliflora [root]), and the *guì zhī* (cinnamon twig) to assist the *fú líng* (poria). *Gān cǎo* (licorice [root]), *shēng jiāng* (ginger), and *dà zǎo* (jujube [fruit]) regulated and harmonized the constructive and defensive [qi] and at the same time moved [the pathogen] to the surface, unblocking the yang to circulate water and induce urination, therefore rapidly dispersing the swelling.

Case 2: *A 24 year-old male*

One case of the use of modified Yuè Bì Tāng
(Spleen-Effusing Decoction) in the treatment of wind water

Initial report: The patient had been suffering from recurrent edematous swelling of the face, head, and extremities for more than a year. In the last year the use of prepared Chinese medicines for strengthening the spleen and enriching the kidney had failed to control his edematous swelling. As the swelling had recurred the patient consulted Master Qin for a diagnosis.

Diagnostic examination: Upon examination it was evident that the edematous swelling was most severe in the upper part of the body, particularly in the head, face, and chest. This was accompanied by thoracic oppression and vexation heat, cough, inability to lie flat, thirst, and no appetite. The flesh of both hands was dry and looked as if it had been soaked in alkaline water and the [patient's] urination was short and yellow. The pulse was deep, wiry, and rapid, while the tongue was clean with a pale body.

Discrimination of patterns. The pattern related to a failure of transportation and transformation within the spleen and a loss of clearing and depuration within the lung.

Treatment methods: Treatment was with modified *Yuè Bì Tāng* (Spleen-Effusing Decoction).

PRESCRIPTION

má huáng	ephedra	3g.
xìng rén	apricot kernel (peeled)	9g.
zǐ sū yè	perilla leaf	5g.
shēng shí gāo	crude gypsum	24g.
fú líng	poria	12g.
tōng cǎo	rice-paper plant pith	3g.

After administration of one dose of the medication there was a frightful cough with expectoration and vomitting of sticky phelgm. This indicated an improvement in the perfusion and free flow of lung qi. Following another two doses the cough became sparse and the chest became relaxed. After another two doses the vexation heat was eliminated and the volume of urine increased. Finally, *Wǔ Pí Sǎn Yǐn* (Five-Peel Powder) combined with *Xiāo Fěn Qīng Yǐn* (Minor Seams-Clearing Beverage) was administered to regulate and rectify.

PRESCRIPTION

sāng bái pí	mulberry root bark
chén pí	tangerine peel
fú líng	poria
dà fù pí	areca husk
zhǐ ké	bitter orange
yì yǐ rén	coix [seed]
xìng rén	apricot kernel

The patient was [thus] cured.

Commentary

According to the *Nèi Jīng*, "swelling above is called wind, while swelling in the legs and shins is called water." In examining the particulars of this case, they are similar to "wind water," although there were no symptoms indicative of an external pathogen, nor was the pulse floating. On the contrary, it was sinking. However, according to the patient, during each episode of the illness, he would first become aware of fullness and oppression in the middle cavity, gradually followed by thoracic pi, shortness of breath, and cough, [all of] which were indicative of "all damp swelling and fullness pertains to the spleen," and [thus] indicated that the root of the illness was in the middle burner.

The upward counterflow of water qi obstructs the lung qi, which becomes depressed and generates heat. Clearing and depurative functions fail to circulate and the fluids cannot be distributed. For this illness, agents were indicated to dry dampness and disinhibit urination, and as there was an upward counterflow, these had to be combined with substances for perfusing the lung and normalizing the qi; thus *Yuè Bì Tāng* (Spleen-Effusing Decoction) was indicated.

Master Qin was extremely skilled in the utilization of medicinals in prescription, and in this case [he] used *má huáng* (ephedra) to open the lung, yet as he didn't want to induce diaphoresis he used a relatively light dose, only three grams. This was assisted by the acrid, fragrant *zǐ sū yè* (perilla leaf), which enters both the lung and spleen channels to diffuse and free the upper burner, as well as dispelling damp turbidity from the middle burner. Again, *shí gāo* (gypsum) and *xìng rén* (apricot kernel) were combined with *má huáng* (ephedra) to diffuse and downbear the lung qi, clear heat, and eliminate vexation. *Fú líng* (poria) and *tōng cǎo* (rice-paper plant pith) blandly percolated and disinhibited the urine.

The prescription was small with only a few carefully considered medicinals yet [it] achieved the result. In this case, the course of the illness was relatively extended. However, there were no obvious symptoms of kidney vacuity and it had not yet involved the lower burner. Therefore, the use of medicinals for enriching the kidney would have been premature and excessive, as well as [having] hindered the circulation of qi and blood.

Case 3. *Wang, a 26 year-old female*

One case of the use of Zhēn Wǔ Tāng (True Warrior Decoction) with additions in the treatment and cure of water swelling and palpitations

Initial report: The patient reported that she had suffered from palpitations and thoracic oppression for more than five years and had most recently experienced edematous swelling in the lower limbs. She consulted Master Qin for a diagnosis.

Diagnostic examination: There was intense edematous swelling in her lumbar region extending to her feet and back, distension and fullness in her abdominal area, nausea and vomiting, palpitations, rough respiration, insomnia, extremely scanty urination, and pasty thin stools. Particularly evident was the cyanosis of the lips and the red-purple tinge to both hands, as well as cheeks [that were so] flushed [that it looked] as if she were wearing makeup. The tip of the tongue was red and the coat was white and slimy, the pulse was fine, rapid, and wiry.

Discrimination of patterns: This pertained to a floating of water due to a vacuity of yang, with a stasis of qi and blood.

Treatment methods: *Zhēn Wǔ Tāng* (True Warrior Deoction) with additions was selected.

PRESCRIPTION

fù zǐ	aconite [accessory tuber], sliced	6g.
shēng jiāng	ginger	6g.
bái zhú	ovate atractylodes [root], fried	9g.
bái sháo yào	white peony [root]	9g.
fú líng	poria	15g.
shā rén	amomum [fruit]	2g.
mù xiāng	saussurea [root]	2g.

The condition calmed down after administration of the medication. After four consecutive administrations of the medication there was an increase in the volume of urine, and the edematous swelling in the lower extremities essentially disappeared, remaining only in the feet and spine. The abdominal distension and vomiting and the nausea also changed for the better, although the flushed cheeks remained along with episodes of irritability. For a time the patient would cough and there would be blood mixed with the phlegm. The pulse was fine and rapid, and not quiet[3] and wiry. The longstanding illness was that of urgent vexation, an unrestrained floating of yang, an upward surge of liver fire attacking the lung. Therefore, there was a bloody cough. The previous prescripiton was adhered to [but] with the deletion of *mù xiāng* (saussurea [root]) and the addition of five grams of *Dài Gé Sǎn* (Indigo and Clamshell Powder). After two doses, the bloody cough was arrested and the condition gradually stabilized.

Commentary

In considering this case, the source [of the illness] was a weakness of heart yang and a failure to warm and transport water dampness from the middle burner. However, the symptoms of the flushed cheeks amply revealed the congestion of qi and water and upward floating of vacuity yang. It was not only a weakness and defeat of stomach qi, there was also a dangerous weakness of heart and kidney yang tending toward vacuity desertion at any [given] time. Therefore, *Zhēn Wǔ Tāng* (True Warrior Decoction) with additions was chosen for therapy. Support of the yang and warming and transforming were primary, asssisted by restraint of the yin and strengthening the spleen. [This succeeded] so that following four doses an obvious effect was realized.

In a patient with excessive floating of vacuity yang such as in the case of an effulgence of liver fire, protection against blood patterns is indicated. In this case there was also a bloody cough due to liver fire attacking the lung, so fragrant drying substances were deleted and those in the class of clearing the liver and settling cough were added. As expected there was a rapid turnaround of the pathomechanism.

Case 4. *Patient Qiu, a 54 year old female*

One case of benefitting the stomach and engendering fluids as the primary treatment and cure of water swelling from vacuity of spleen and stomach

Initial report: As a result of going bathing and then contracting a chill, edematous swelling appeared in the lower limbs. The condition gradually increased in intensity as a result of her attention to her daily household duties. [When] the illness had persisted for nine months, she consulted Master Qin for a diagnosis.

---

[3]Trans: "Not quiet," *bù qīng ān,* refers to a sense of reverberation in addition to the wiriness.

Diagnostic examination: Edematous swelling with pitting upon palpation was evident over the entire body, with numbness of the hands, a frightened and confused mental state, a dry mouth, and desire for fluids. [She experienced] a sense of hunger [in her abdomen] and ate more than usual. [Her] urine was copious and clear; [her] bowel movements were normal. The pulse was wiry, large, and rapid, while the tongue was glossy red and cracked. The facial complexion was withered yellow and lusterless.

Discrimination of patterns and treatment methods: The root was the insufficiency of fluids in the spleen and stomach and so the treatment focused on methods for benefitting the stomach and engendering fluids.

PRESCRIPTION

shí hú	dendrobium [stem]	12g.
běi shā shēn	glehnia [root]	12g.
tiān huā fěn	trichosanthes root	12g.
bái sháo yào	white peony [root]	12g.
shān yào	dioscorea [root]	24g.
huáng qí	astragalus [root]	10g.
bái zhú	ovate atractylodes [root]	10g.
mài mén dōng	ophiopogon [tuber]	10g.
yì yǐ rén	raw coix [seed]	15g.
chì xiǎo dòu	rice bean	30g.

After administration of three doses of the medication, the swelling gradually abated. After six doses, the redness in the tongue also paled and a thin coat developed.

Commentary

This case of edematous swelling of more than nine months duration is [an example of a] mixed vacuity and repletion. Master Qin captured the primary pattern within the many complexities of the symptoms and established the principal pathomechanism. Of chief consideration was the vacuity of the spleen which failed to transform dampness. The *Nèi Jīng* states: "all damp swelling and fullness pertains to the spleen." However, other than the manifestations of spleen vacuity and an insufficiency of generation and transformation such as [evidenced by] the withered yellow facial complexion, [symptoms such as] the numb hands and palpitations, the symptoms of thirst and capacity for drinking, hunger and increased appetite, and long clear urination failed to tally with a pathomechanism of damp hindrance. On the contrary, the tongue and pulse were expressions of an extreme vacuity of fluids within the spleen and stomach. Therefore, he relied upon the statement of Huà Xiùyún:

> *In an insufficiency of spleen yang, with damp cold in the stomach, where warming, drying, upbearing, and transporting are indicated for viscera and bowels alike, then naturally abide scrupulously by Dōngyuán's [treatment] methods. But if the spleen yang is not depleted, and there is a dry fire within the stomach, then naturally we abide by Master Chi's methods for nourishing the stomach.*

Therefore this case is an example of water swelling that is primarily due to a relatively unusual vacuity of yin in the spleen and stomach. The primary treatment was toward benefitting the stomach and generating fluids, and so a satisfactory result as achieved.

(The above was arranged by Dú Huáitáng [a disciple of Qin].)

BIBLIOGRAPHY

Chinese Sources

Qin Bo-wei Yi Wen Ji (The Collected Medical Writings of Qin Bo-wei). Hunan, China: Hunan Science and Technology Press, 1981.

Dong Jian Hua et al., eds. Zhong Guo Xian Dai Ming Zhong Yi Yi An Jing Hua (The Essential Case Histories of China's Famous Chinese Medical Physicians. Beijing, China: Beijing Press, 1990.

Wiseman Nigel. English-Chinese–Chinese-English Dictionary of Chinese Medicine. Hunan, China: Hunan Science and Technology Press, 1995.

Peng Huai Ren et al., eds. Zhong Hua Ming Yi Fang Ji Da Quan (A Complete Compendium of Famous Chinese Herbal Prescriptions). China: Jin dun Press, 1990.

Jiangsu College of New Medicine, eds. Zhong Yao Da Ci Dian (The Encyclopedia of Chinese Medicinals). Shanghai, China: Shanghai Science and Technology Press, 1990.

English Sources

Chace Charles. Fleshing Out the Bones, Case Histories in the Practice of Chinese Medicine. Boulder, CO: Blue Poppy Press, 1992.

INDEX

P

pài jiāng: 139

Pain and Diarrhea Formula: 53, 60

pain in the chest: 14

pain in the eye: 28, 71

pain in the joints: 14

pain in the lumbar spine: 26

pain of the abdominal cavity: 79

pain upon palpation: 124

pale menses: 10

pale tongue body: 10

pallid complexion: 23, 169

palpitations: 13, 18, 45, 47, 55, 95, 155, 168, 185, 187-190, 196, 198

pàng dà hài: 93, 114, 151, 153

panting [dyspnea]: 14, 35, 153, 168

pào jiāng: 51, 65, 134, 136, 184

paralysis: 15, 86, 167

paranoia: 10

parasite accumulation patterns: 22

parotitis with chills and fever: 120

pasty stools: 143

pathogenic cold: 19, 38, 41, 43, 56, 63, 67

pathogenic heat: 45-46, 48, 67, 81, 125, 133

pathogenic heat with cardiac vexation and agitation: 81

pathogenic warm heat: 46

pathogenic wind: 88, 182

peach kernel: 34, 58, 72, 74-75, 108, 134-135, 139, 156, 193

Peach Kernel Qi-Infusing Decoction: 134

pear peel: 119

pearl: 46-47, 85, 88-89

pearl Margarita: 46-47, 85, 88-89

pearly sweat: 20

pediatric gan accumulation: 137

pediatric measles: 131, 154

pèi lán: 108, 192

péng é zhú: 74

peony [root]: 6, 16, 30, 35-38, 42-46, 48-54, 56, 58, 60, 62-66, 69-73, 75, 77, 81, 89, 97, 100-101, 103-105, 111, 121-122, 124, 127-129, 133-134, 136, 139-140, 144, 176, 182, 184, 188, 193, 197-198

pepper: 6

Perfect Major Supplementation Decoction: 84

Perfect Major Supplementation Pill: 170

perfusing the qi: 151

perfusion: 176, 195

peridontitis with chills and fever: 120

perilla leaf: 49-50, 78, 93, 118, 126, 151, 153, 195-196

perilla stem: 34-35

periumbilical area: 26-27

persimmon calyx: 104

perspiration of the head: 131, 167-168

peucedanum [root]: 79, 93, 105, 129, 138, 151-152, 182, 190

phellodendron [bark]: 55, 57, 104, 106, 123, 127, 136

phlegm dampness: 50, 59, 191

phlegm depression: 14

phlegm fire: 51

phlegm malaria: 138

phlegm rheum: 24, 102, 105, 168

phlegm turbidity: 149-150

phlegmatic cough: 108, 182

phlegmatic respiration: 20-21

phlegm-dampness: 151

photophobia: 17-18

phragmites [root]: 54-55, 96, 108, 113, 118, 152, 178, 192-193

pi: 13, 15, 22-23, 36, 40, 87, 104, 107, 125, 195

pi fullness distension: 22

pi oppression: 40

pí pá yè: 36, 96, 153

Pí Yuē Má Rén Wán: 124

pǐ kuài: 22

pǐ qì: 21, 22

pig's bile: 124

Pinella, Unripe Bitter Orange and Ovate Atractylodes Pill: 110

pinellia [tuber]: 34, 47-49, 51, 58, 61, 93, 98, 103, 105-106, 110-111, 114, 125-126, 130, 135-136, 138, 142, 151, 176-177, 182, 191

Píng Wèi Sǎn: 106

placenta: 169

plantago seed: 54, 63, 65

platycodon [root]: 93, 97, 105, 113, 118, 120, 126-128, 139-141, 151-153, 176, 182

plum pit qi: 28

plum seed qi: 28

pneumonia: 8, 193

polygala [root]: 144, 167, 185-186, 188-189

polyporus: 177

poppy husk: 97-98

poor digestion: 12-13, 36, 119

poria: 34, 44-46, 49, 51-52, 57, 61-62, 64-66, 78, 93, 97, 100, 105-107, 126, 128, 134, 136-139, 144, 165-168, 176-177, 182, 186, 189, 193-197

Poria (Hoelen), Licorice, Schisandra, Ginger, and Asarum Decoction: 105

postprandial discomfort: 188

postprandial distension: 27, 194

postprandial cardiac pain: 190

postpartum hemmorrhage: 85

precipitation: 27, 124-125, 127, 146, 179

precordial pain: 186-189

pregnancy epilepsy: 88

prepared rehmannia [root]: 100-101

pressing pain anterior and posterior to the ear: 120

primary treatment: 44, 76, 98, 100, 110, 197-198

processed honey: 124

production of heat in the stomach and intestines: 145

production of qi: 56

prolapse of the anus: 20

promote the exterior: 121

promoting appetite: 171

promoting diaphoresis: 151

promoting the generation of blood: 72

pronounced abdominal distension: 22

protect liver yin: 45, 50

protecting the yin: 124

prunella [spike]: 36, 43, 63, 65, 81-83, 96

psoralea [seed]: 169

pú huáng: 70, 186

Pǔ Jì Xiāo Dú Yǐn: 140

puccoon: 130

Pueraria Decoction: 120, 128, 144

pueraria [root]: 61, 79, 97, 116, 120, 128-129, 132, 139, 144